RISE™

The Beginning of Balance

The RISE™ Framework for Whole-Being Wellness

Rooted • Intentional • Strong • Energized

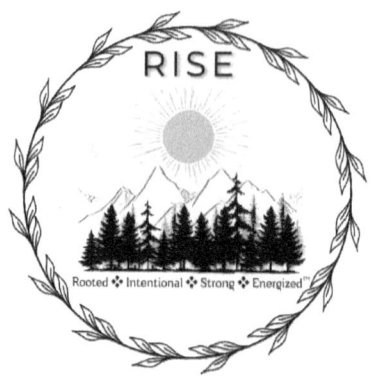

A transformational book series exploring balance, belief, and embodied wellness.

Books in the Series

RISE™ Wellness Journal—Rooted, Intentional, Strong, Energized: Embrace One Year of Habits, Healing, and Hope

RISE™ The Beginning of Balance—How Rooted, Intentional, Strong, and Energized Living Transforms the Whole Self: A Framework for Whole-Being Wellness

The Beginning of Balance Chronicles: The Lived Record of Learning to Inhabit RISE

Explore all titles and resources at HealthyInHeart.com

RISE™

The Beginning of Balance

~

How Rooted, Intentional, Strong, and Energized

Living Transforms the Whole Self—

A Framework for Whole-Being Wellness

Angel Tate Keaton

Healthy in Heart Media™, LLC
Roanoke, VA

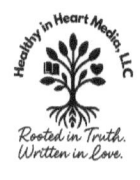

prescribe the use of any technique as a form of treatment for medical, emotional, psychological, or physical conditions without the guidance of a licensed physician or qualified healthcare provider, either directly or indirectly. The intent of the author is solely to offer information of a general nature to support you in your personal journey toward emotional, physical, mental, and spiritual well-being.

If you choose to apply any of the information presented in this book, you do so of your own volition. The author and the publisher assume no responsibility for your actions or any consequences that may arise from the use or misuse of the information contained herein.

No Guarantee of Outcomes
The practices and concepts presented in this book are intended to support whole-being wellness. Individual experiences and results may vary. The author and publisher make no guarantees regarding any specific physical, emotional, or spiritual outcomes resulting from the application of this material.

Educational Purpose Notice
This book is provided for general informational and educational purposes only and is not intended as a substitute for professional medical, psychological, counseling, or therapeutic care.

Emergency Help Notice
This material is not intended for crises. If you are experiencing a medical, mental-health, or safety emergency, contact local emergency services or a licensed professional immediately.

No Professional Relationship Notice
Reading this book does not establish a counseling, coaching, therapeutic, or professional relationship between the reader and the author or publisher. This material is for personal growth and educational use only and is not a substitute for individualized professional advice, diagnosis, or treatment.

Dedication

For my **Mama**,
whose quiet faith and steady strength taught me
that love still grows
even in hard soil.

For **my sister, Pamela,**
Whose struggle taught me compassion,
And whose story reminds me why rising matters.

For **every woman.**
who has learned to find her voice, and to live free,
who chooses to break the cycle,
who refuses to return to what broke her,
who realizes that freedom begins
the moment she believes she's worthy of it.
Rising is not easy—but it is sacred.
May your rising be the healing of generations.

For **Todd**,
my safe place,
my encourager,
and the one who reminds me to rest when I forget how.

And for **you**—
the one still learning to breathe between striving and surrender,
the one still trying to believe that healing is possible,
and needing to remember that wholeness is never about perfection.
May you rise again and again,
until your life becomes a rhythm of grace.

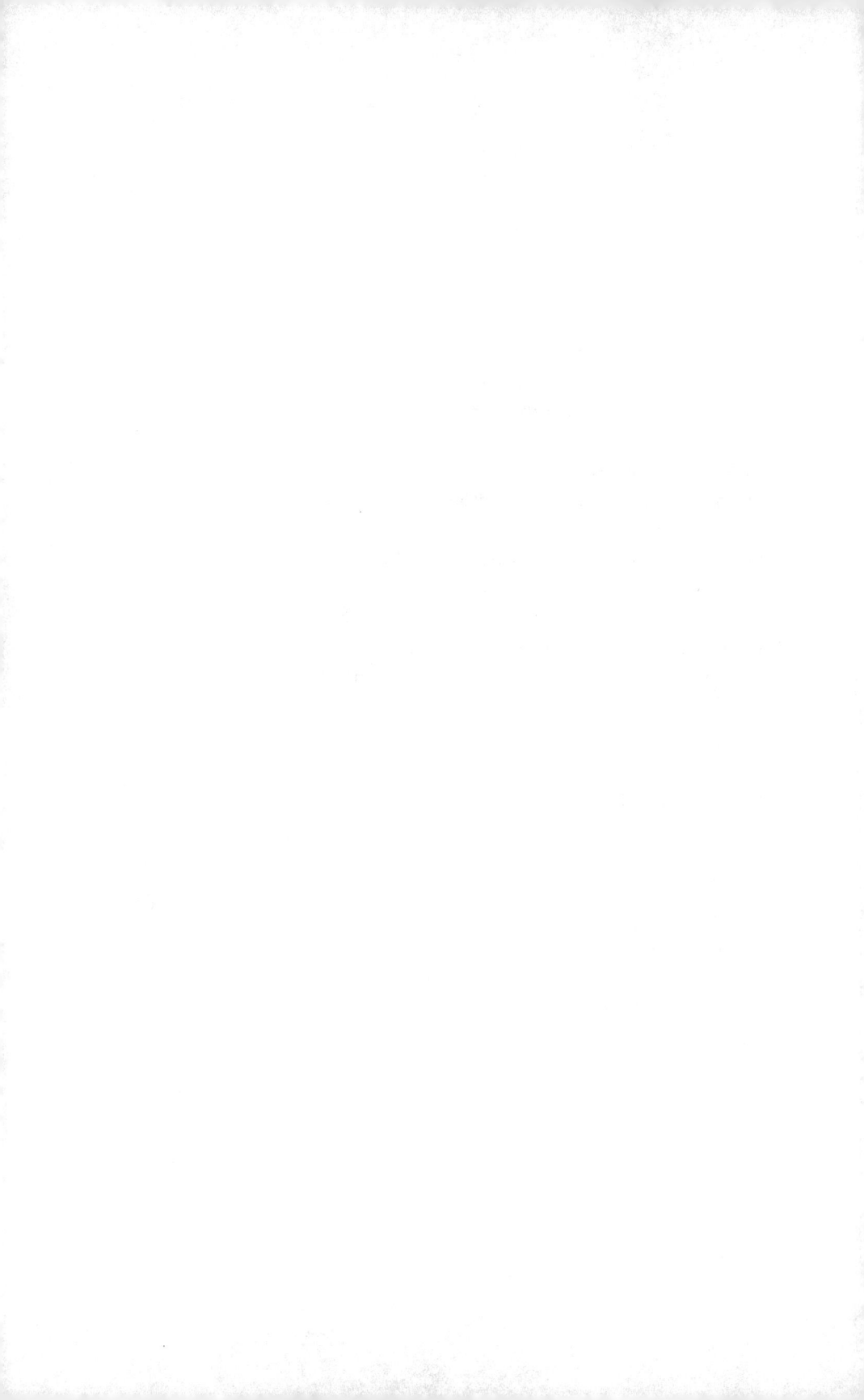

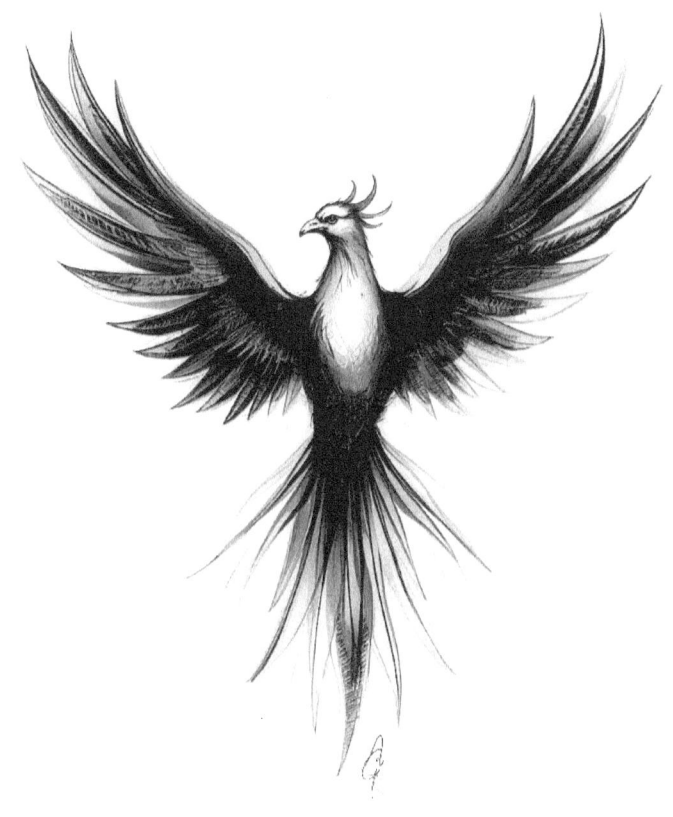

When the phoenix burns,
It does not perish.
It rises—refined.

For everything there is a season,

and a time for every purpose under heaven.

Ecclesiastes 3:1

Table of Contents

Preface — Why I Wrote This Book

When I first began writing this book, I didn't set out to create a wellness philosophy.

I set out to survive.

Not the kind of survival where you're clinging to life after a car crash or a hurricane—though sometimes it felt like that.

This was the slow kind.

The kind where you wake up each morning already exhausted, where your body aches for reasons the doctors can't explain, and your spirit whispers, *"There has to be more than this."*

For years, I lived in cycles of striving—trying to be healthier, holier, thinner, better. I read every diet book, listened to every podcast, and chased every new promise of transformation. Yet underneath it all was the same ache. I didn't want another plan. I wanted peace.

That longing became the seed for RISE: The Beginning of Balance.

The Turning Point

My story isn't tidy.

It's marked with trauma, loss, disordered eating, and decades of believing that healing was for other people. I carried the inherited scripts of my upbringing—faith mixed with fear, devotion tangled with perfectionism.

I grew up in a Pentecostal Holiness world where women's worth was measured by modesty and obedience. I learned early to cover up—to hide my skin, my voice, my questions. My mother's quiet shame over her darker skin taught me that even the color of your body could be a source of shame. My siblings' teasing taught me that my size was something I needed to apologize for.

The first "diet" I ever went on was at age twelve, prescribed by a family doctor who told me to eat tuna fish for every single meal. My earliest memories of food are filled with both comfort and condemnation. Food became both a friend that soothed me and an enemy that betrayed me.

By adulthood, I was living in the full weight of that war—body, mind, and spirit disconnected.

Every health crisis I faced—Type II diabetes, hypertension, obesity, and even a rash that covered 90 percent of my body—became both symptom and teacher.

When medication lists grew longer, and hope grew shorter, I finally admitted: the system wasn't working.

The medical model wanted to manage my symptoms; I wanted to understand their cause.

And beneath it all, I sensed something sacred whispering: There is another way.

When Healing Found Me

Healing didn't come as a lightning bolt of revelation. It came through ordinary moments of grace.

Through mentors like Karen Smith, who taught me to see the body as an ecosystem rather than a machine, to listen to the language of my cells and the stories my emotions told.

Through teachers like Ross K. Nichols, who challenged me to question everything I'd inherited and seek truth beyond tradition.

Through voices like Dr. John McDougall, Dr. Neal Barnard, Dr. Caldwell Esselstyn, and Dr. Alan Goldhammer, who taught me that food is more than fuel—it's communication.

Through the memory of my Cherokee ancestors' wisdom, I am reminded to honor plants as partners in healing, not commodities to be consumed.

These experiences formed threads of a tapestry that I didn't know I was weaving. Each one whispered a single truth: the body, mind, and spirit were never meant to live in separate rooms.

Healing isn't about conquering disease—it's about coming back into rhythm with life itself.

The Ache for Wholeness

For most of my life, I thought "health" was about control. Calories, numbers, metrics, achievements. I thought discipline would fix me.

But the more I tried to control my body, the more it rebelled.

I dieted, I binged, I fasted for all the wrong reasons. I prayed, repented, and punished myself for not being "spiritual enough," and would my body just be healed and thin already?

And then something shifted.

In the stillness after burnout, I heard a softer invitation—not to strive, but to listen.

- o Listen to the body that had carried me through every storm.
- o Listen to the spirit that had never stopped reaching for hope.
- o Listen to the rhythms of creation that pulsed all around me.

That listening became language.

That language became a framework.

And that framework became RISE.

Why Balance Matters

For too long, we've been taught to live at extremes—to chase productivity until collapse, to heal only when broken, to seek rest only when sick.

Balance, in our culture, is treated like a luxury—something you earn only after you've proven your worth through exhaustion.

But creation itself tells another story.

From the first sunrise in Genesis, everything sacred follows a rhythm of work and rest, light and dark, inhale and exhale.

Even our biology echoes that truth—our hearts beat in patterns, our hormones rise and fall in circadian rhythm, our cells regenerate in nightly cycles of renewal.

When we step out of that rhythm, we break down—not just physically, but emotionally and spiritually.

Balance isn't optional—it's design.

RISE was born to help us remember that design and live in harmony with it again.

From Perfection to Presence

When I began forming RISE, I sought a framework that would honor both science and soul, blending modern psychology with ancient wisdom.

But as I wrote, something unexpected happened: I realized that I was still chasing perfection, even in my attempt to teach balance.

So, I stopped trying to write a manual for transformation.

Instead, I wrote a mirror—a reflection of what it means to live imperfectly but intentionally.

This book isn't a checklist; it's a conversation.

It's not about mastering wellness; it's about making peace with your humanity.

RISE doesn't demand that you become more—it invites you to become whole.

What RISE Really Means

Each letter of RISE carries a truth that saved my life:

- o **Rooted** — in identity, faith, and the quiet knowing that you belong here.
- o **Intentional** — choosing presence over autopilot and awareness over avoidance.
- o **Strong** — not through force, but through surrender, boundaries, and grace.
- o **Energized** — living in rhythm with creation, not in resistance to it.

These four words are not steps to climb but anchors to return to.

They are reminders that you are a whole being—physical, emotional, mental, and spiritual—and all four dimensions deserve care.

Why I Had to Write This

I wrote this book because I got tired of seeing people—especially women—measure their worth by weight scales, productivity charts, or spiritual performance.

I wrote it because I know what it feels like to live disconnected from your body, to believe that rest is lazy, that grace is weakness, that slowing down means falling behind.

I wrote it because I wanted to tell the truth:

You can't hate yourself into healing.

You can't strive your way into peace.

You can't compartmentalize your way into wholeness.

I wrote it because I needed to read it.

And when I finally began to live what I was writing—when I stopped chasing perfection and started cultivating rhythm—everything changed.

My health improved.

My relationships deepened.

My joy returned.

But most importantly, my faith expanded.

I began to see God not as a distant judge tallying my failures, but as the Gardener inviting me back into the soil of balance and belonging.

That is what this book is: an invitation back to the Garden within you.

A Philosophy of Whole-Being Living

The RISE framework isn't another "wellness trend."

It is a reclaiming.

It reclaims what modern life has divided: body from soul, doing from being, striving from surrender.

It's a reminder that wellness isn't one-dimensional—it's whole-being wellness.

And whole-being wellness requires both grounding and grace, science and Spirit, discipline and delight.

This book is the first in a series that explores how to live that integration daily.

It's the beginning of balance, not the final word on it.

Each page is a stepping-stone toward your own understanding of what it means to live rooted, intentional, strong, and energized.

To the Reader Who Is Tired

If you're reading this with weary eyes and an overfull heart, I want you to know: I see you.

If you've tried every plan and still feel lost, this book is for you.

If you've spent your life caring for others but forgotten how to care for yourself, this book is for you.

If you've believed that balance is for people with more time, more money, or more willpower—this book is especially for you.

You don't have to earn balance.

You just have to remember it.

You were designed for rhythm.

For rest.

For renewal.

And that remembering begins here—one breath, one truth, one chapter at a time.

Why I Still Believe in Beginning

When I look back over my life—the trauma, the weight, the loss, the rebuilding—I can trace a thread of grace through it all.

Every detour taught me something vital about the human condition and the divine compassion woven through it.

Every failure was a falling forward into greater wisdom.

If I could tell you one thing before you turn the page, it would be this:

Don't despise your beginnings.

Beginnings are sacred ground.

Beginnings are where potential meets possibility.

They're where you finally stop running and decide to root.

RISE isn't about reinventing yourself; it's about re-inhabiting yourself.

Coming home to your body.

Coming home to your truth.

Coming home to the balance you were created for.

That's why I wrote this book.

Because somewhere between faith and fatigue, I found the rhythm that holds them both.

And I believe you can too.

A Final Word Before We Begin

You don't need to have it all figured out.

You don't need to be ready in the perfect sense of the word.

You just need to be willing—to be curious, compassionate, and open.

This book won't demand anything from you that you don't already have within you.

It will simply remind you of what's been waiting all along.

So, take a deep breath.

Release the tension in your shoulders.

Let the striving soften.

You're not stepping into another self-help project.

You're stepping into presence.

And presence—that sacred, embodied, everyday awareness—is where balance truly begins.

Welcome home.

Welcome to RISE.

Welcome to The Beginning of Balance.

Acknowledgments

When I look back on the path that led me to write *RISE*^{TM} *The Beginning of Balance*, I can see that it wasn't written in isolation. Every chapter, every revelation, every quiet moment of surrender came through the influence, encouragement, and wisdom of others. This book may carry my name on the cover, but it carries our fingerprints on every page.

My Heavenly Father

First and always, I give thanks to my Creator—GOD—for the breath of life, the lessons of grace, and the constant rhythm of mercy that never ceases. Every truth written here was first whispered through prayer, silence, and the gentle leading of His Spirit.

Without Your guidance, Father, there would be no RISE. There would be no me.

You are the origin of balance itself—the still point in every storm.

May this work reflect Your heartbeat of restoration and remind all who read it that You are not a God of chaos but of order, peace, and wholeness.

My Husband, Todd

To my very best, most faithful friend and greatest earthly supporter, Todd—thank you for believing in me when I didn't yet believe in myself.

You have been patient through every late-night writing session, every moment of doubt, every new "big idea" I couldn't stop talking about. You listened when I needed to vent, you steadied me when I felt overwhelmed, and you celebrated every small victory as if it were your own.

Thank you for encouraging me to follow the call that GOD placed on my life and for reminding me to rest when I tried to pour from an empty cup.

You have shown me what partnership truly means: two people walking in rhythm with one heart.

This book—and this life—would not exist without your love.

My Family

To my daughter, Kelsey—thank you for teaching me that love requires both grounding and grace. You remind me daily that healing isn't something we pass down—it's something we model.

To my dear mother—thank you for your strength, for your prayers, and for the faith that shaped my earliest understanding of God. Though you've walked through storms and unhealed generations, your perseverance taught me to rise again and again.

To my father, whose memory lives on in every lesson about hard work and compassion—thank you for showing me what it means to keep going even when the path is unclear.

To my sisters and brother, and especially to my late sister, whose loss still ripples through my heart—you are part of this story, too. The pain, the laughter, the rebuilding—it all lives here, redeemed through prayer, if not through repentance.

Karen Smith, My Teacher and Friend

Karen, you were the first person who saw something in me that I could not yet see in myself. You taught me to listen to my inner wisdom and to trust the voice of my body as a messenger, not an enemy.

Your mentorship planted the seeds that grew into the RISE framework. From you, I learned that health is not achieved through punishment but through partnership with my body. You modeled gentleness, curiosity, and courage in a world obsessed with control.

This book carries your imprint in every mention of intuition, balance, and embodied truth. Thank you for lighting the first candle that helped me find my way home.

Ross K. Nichols, My Teacher and Friend

Ross, thank you for teaching me the sacred art of inquiry—for showing me that faith deepens, not weakens, when we dare to question.

Your work taught me that truth does not fear examination and that the journey of seeking is, in itself, holy. Your willingness to ask the hard questions gave me permission to do the same and to keep asking until belief and evidence stood in harmony. Because of you, I learned that living in alignment means letting go of dogma and embracing the deeper rhythm of discovery.

All the Voices That Shaped My Understanding

To Dr. John McDougall, Dr. Caldwell Esselstyn, Dr. T. Colin Campbell, Dr. Neal Barnard, Dr. Doug Lisle, and Dr. Alan

Goldhammer—thank you for pioneering the evidence that what we eat, breathe, and believe truly shapes our lives.

Your research and teachings gave me the language to describe what I had already begun to experience: that the body longs for harmony, and when given the chance, it will heal itself.

To Dr. John Bergman—thank you for opening my eyes to the chemicals and environmental toxins we unknowingly accept as "normal" today. Your work reminded me that we are whole beings, not a collection of parts.

You each gave me pieces of the puzzle that became the foundation for RISE—where science meets sacred design.

My Native American Ancestors

To the women who came before me—my mother, grandmother, and all those unnamed but felt through memory—thank you for the wisdom you carried in your hands and hearts.

You taught me to respect the earth that feeds us, to use the whole plant and not just its parts, and to leave something behind for the next generation.

Your teachings echo in every garden metaphor I use and in every reminder to honor creation as teacher.

Your reverence for balance, reciprocity, and rhythm shaped the heart of this philosophy long before I gave it words.

The Early RISE with Momentum Circle Members

To the first brave souls who joined me in the earliest RISE Circle—you are the living proof that community heals what isolation cannot.

You show up week after week, share your stories with honesty, and create a space where everyone can exhale. Your vulnerability made this movement real.

You reminded me that healing is not a solo pursuit—it's a shared rhythm. Each of you holds a piece of this circle's heart, and I am endlessly grateful for your courage to begin before everything made sense.

Thank you for trusting the process, for speaking truth, and for helping me refine RISE into something that could hold all of us.

The Readers and Future Leaders of RISE

If you are holding this book in your hands, you are part of this story now.

You are the continuation of this work, the next ripple in the movement toward wholeness.

Thank you for reading with an open heart, for reflecting honestly, for daring to believe that balance is possible even here, even now.

Your willingness to begin again—to root, to rise, to realign—changes more than you can imagine.

It changes families, communities, and legacies.

My prayer for you is that you will not only read these words but live them.

That you will walk this path with curiosity and kindness toward yourself.

That you will start small, begin again, and keep going.

Because the world needs your rhythm.

The world needs your light.

The world needs you—whole, not perfect.

And Finally — You, the Reader

This is more than acknowledgment—it's a blessing.

May the pages you've read become pathways of peace.

May the truths you've uncovered settle softly in your spirit.

May you feel seen, safe, and strengthened by the rhythm of your own becoming.

May you rise when life asks you to,

> Rest when your soul requires it,

> And remember—balance isn't somewhere you arrive;

> It's how you live along the way.

Thank you for walking this road with me. Thank you for bringing your story to the circle. And thank you for reminding me, again and again, that the greatest transformations happen when we rise together.

With all my heart,

Angel

A Note to the Reader

This book is not meant to be rushed.

It was written to be *walked through*—slowly, intentionally, and with the same grace you'll be invited to give yourself.

RISE™ *The Beginning of Balance* is more than a framework; it's a rhythm. You'll notice that the chapters move like breath: inhale truth, exhale application, rest in reflection. Some sections will evoke emotion or memory; others will require quiet. That is the design. Growth doesn't happen in straight lines—it unfolds in seasons.

Throughout these pages, you'll find reflection prompts and simple practices. They are not assignments to complete but invitations to notice. You can write in a journal, record your thoughts, or simply pause and sit with what rises. The goal is not mastery — it's awareness.

You may come to this book seeking health, peace, purpose, or connection. Wherever you are, begin there. The path of balance always starts at the point of noticing: *I am ready to live differently.*

Each concept—Rooted, Intentional, Strong, and Energized—builds upon the others. Together, they create a circle of wholeness that honors your mind, body, emotions, and spirit as one integrated system.

You will also see language drawn from both science, spirituality, psychology, and practice. The RISE philosophy welcomes all who long to live more consciously, regardless of their spiritual or philosophical background. I hope that you will feel at home here.

Take your time. Breathe often. Let the words settle. And when life feels too loud, return to this truth:

You are already in the process of becoming whole.

Not because you've achieved balance, but because you are brave enough to seek it.

Overview of the RISE Framework

A Pathway Back to Whole-Being Wellness

RISE is more than a wellness model — it is a way of returning to internal balance, where every part of you can breathe again.

Rooted, Intentional, Strong, and Energized.

When people rise, they rise in four dimensions — body, mind, spirit, and community — each supporting the other like threads in a tapestry of wholeness.

The Beginning of Balance volume guides you into equilibrium — learning to create harmony between your pace, your priorities, your emotions, and your daily choices.

Before habits become sustainable, balance must be restored.

RISE offers language, symbols, and gentle practices that help you steady your life one small shift at a time.

Below is the complete framework.

R — Rooted

Rooted people are steady, grounded, nourished, and connected.

Labels, storms, or circumstances do not define them, because their identity is anchored in something deeper and more eternal.

Being rooted means:

> Strong internal foundations

Eating what nourishes

Slowing down enough to listen

Living from truth, not reaction

Returning to who you are beneath old labels

Rootedness is the soil where balance begins.

I — Intentional

Intentional living means moving through the world with clarity, purpose, and conscious choice.

It is the opposite of living on autopilot or from inherited beliefs.

Intentionality expresses itself as:

Mindfulness

Choosing rather than drifting

Creating rhythms instead of reacting

Speaking truth with compassion

Aligning actions with values

Intentionality restores balance one decision at a time.

S — Strong

Strength in this journey looks like emotional steadiness, integrity, and internal resilience.

It is the capacity to remain centered even when life becomes imbalanced.

It is the ability to stay centered in truth even when circumstances shake.

This dimension includes:

Emotional strength

Boundaries

Courage

Resilience

Balanced confidence

Willingness to grow

Strength keeps your balance steady when life wobbles.

E — Energized

Energized living is balanced living — not frantic, not depleted.

It is sustainable vitality born from nourishing rhythms and inner alignment.

Energized people experience:

Joy that flows without force

Healthy rhythms of work and rest

Clarity instead of exhaustion

Purpose without burnout

A sense of internal lightness

Energy naturally rises when life is in balance.

The Circle of Wholeness Model

A Whole-System View of Human Flourishing

The Circle of Wholeness is the visual framework that holds the entire RISE model.

It teaches that wellness is not linear — it is circular, interconnected, and dynamic.

> Every area of life affects balance.

> Small shifts ripple into the whole.

> Minor changes create meaningful healing.

> You cannot steady one area without influencing the rest.

The Circle of Wholeness includes Nine Anchors, each represented by a nature-based symbol.

These symbols are simple, universal, and spiritually resonant, so you can explore balance in a way that fits your own rhythm and daily life.

The next page gives you a simple overview of the nine-anchor ecosystem you'll revisit throughout this book.

Introduction: Returning to Rhythm

There is a moment in every healing journey when you realize you're not simply trying to "get better." You're trying to come home — to your body, to your peace, to yourself.

That moment came quietly for me, somewhere between exhaustion and awakening. I had been chasing health for decades — dieting, striving, praying, studying, and searching for answers to questions that kept changing shape. I didn't know then that what I was really searching for wasn't another plan or protocol. It was balance.

Not the kind of balance you can measure on a scale or find in a planner. The kind of balance that lives deep inside — the still point between doing and being, between belief and embodiment. The kind of balance that whispers, you were never broken; you were only disconnected.

For much of my life, I equated wellness with performance: eating perfectly, exercising enough, thinking positively, praying hard, serving more, fixing everything I thought was wrong with me. But no matter how hard I tried, peace remained just out of reach. My body was tired, my emotions scattered, my mind noisy, and my spirit weary.

Eventually, I began to understand that what I called "discipline" was often just fear wearing a holy face — fear of failure, fear of rejection, fear of not being enough. What I needed wasn't more effort; what I needed was alignment.

That realization didn't come all at once. It unfolded slowly — through illness, mentorship, loss, prayer, study, and community. Along the way, I began noticing patterns — not just in my own life, but in those around me. We were all living fragmented stories: one part of us striving, another part hiding, another crying for rest.

RISE was born out of those patterns — out of the recognition that wholeness can only happen when every part of us is allowed to belong.

How RISE Was Born

RISE isn't a quick fix or a one-size-fits-all method. It's a framework — a rhythm — that emerged through years of personal healing, spiritual rediscovery, and walking alongside others who were tired of the endless cycle of self-improvement without self-acceptance.

The name itself — Rooted, Intentional, Strong, Energized — came to me during a season of deep reflection. Each word represented something I had been missing, and something I saw missing in the modern wellness world.

We are taught to hustle, to optimize, to be endlessly productive. But few of us are taught to pause. To listen. To root. To align our daily habits with the deeper rhythms of our biology and the wisdom of our spirit.

The more I studied psychology, faith, and physiology, the clearer it became: imbalance isn't just emotional or spiritual — it's biological. Our bodies and minds are constantly communicating, but modern life has drowned out their conversation.

RISE became my way of restoring that dialogue — a living model for whole-being wellness that unites science and spirit, mindset and movement, breath and belief.

What You'll Discover in These Pages

This book is divided into six parts, each reflecting a stage of the journey from disconnection to integration.

Part I: The Story Behind the Balance — my personal journey of illness, awakening, and mentorship that gave birth to the RISE framework.

Part II: The Longing for Balance — why we crave wholeness, how imbalance shows up, and what it costs us to live divided.

Part III: The Framework of Wholeness — an in-depth look at the four anchors: Rooted, Intentional, Strong, and Energized.

Part IV: The Rhythm of Renewal — how the RISE Circle mirrors the biological rhythms of life — daily, weekly, seasonal, and lifelong.

Part V: Embodiment and Community — how healing deepens when shared in safe, authentic spaces.

Part VI: Integration and Invitation — how to live dynamically in the flow of balance rather than chasing perfection.

Every chapter closes with a Reflection Prompt — a question designed to help you move from reading into living.

This isn't a book to consume; it's an experience to practice. I recommend reading slowly. Keep a journal nearby. When a question stirs you, don't rush to answer it — sit with it. Let your nervous system catch up to your insight. Healing moves at the pace of safety, not speed.

The RISE framework is both scientific and spiritual. You'll find references to circadian rhythm, nutrition, and nervous system regulation right alongside reflections on purpose, presence, and grace because you are both body and soul, form and breath.

You'll also find that this book doesn't demand belief; it invites curiosity. It's written for anyone longing for balance — whether you express that longing through prayer, mindfulness, or a quiet walk in the garden.

My goal is not to tell you what to believe, but to walk with you as you discover truth for yourself — to help you reconnect with the wisdom already planted within you. Because when we learn to listen inwardly, the path toward wholeness reveals itself in its own time and way.

The Beginning of Balance

RISE isn't about rising above life — it's about rising within it.

It's not about escaping the chaos but finding the calm that exists beneath it.

It's not about achieving balance once and for all but learning to return to it again and again.

The rhythm of balance is already within you — waiting to be remembered.

As you move through these pages, may you begin to feel it: in your breath, in your choices, in your pace, and in your peace, because balance isn't something you earn. It's something you remember.

And remembering is how we rise.

PART - I

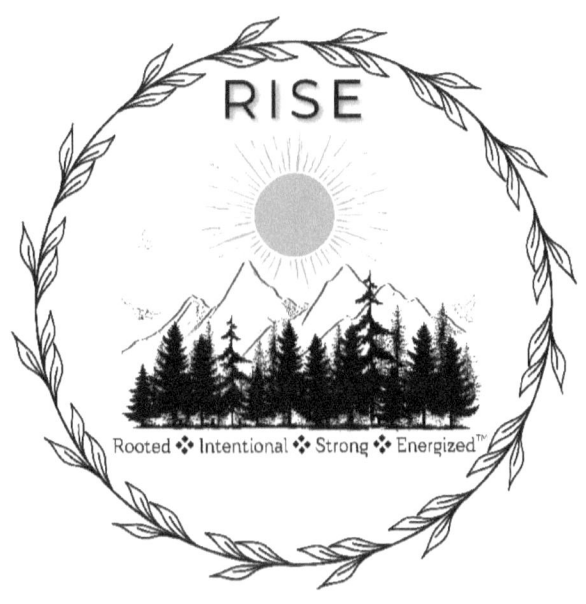

The Story Behind the Balance

Every movement begins with a story, and RISE began with a woman who refused to stay unwell in body, mind, or spirit. My journey toward whole-being wellness did not start with success; it began with shame, exhaustion, and a deep-seated longing to be free. I grew up in the narrow world of Pentecostal Holiness, where holiness was measured by hemlines and hair length. We meant well, but the rules wrapped tighter than the faith beneath them. I learned early that belonging could vanish with one wrong choice of clothing or layer of lipstick. The seeds of body shame were planted before I ever learned self-acceptance.

Pain became my earliest teacher—family ridicule, diet culture, and the belief that thinness equaled worth. Trauma and restriction grew into binge eating and a lifetime of searching for peace inside my own skin. Yet even then, the Creator was weaving purpose through the pain. Through mentors, study, and relentless curiosity, I began collecting fragments of truth: eight years of classes in psychology taught me how the mind works; a healer who showed me that food can harm or heal; and teachers who urged me to question everything.

The years that followed became an education in both science and spirit. From every season of loss and every experiment in health, a pattern began to form—a rhythm of being **Rooted, Intentional, Strong, and Energized.** That rhythm is what eventually became RISE. This first part of the book tells that story: the imperfect beginning, the mentors and mistakes, the long road from survival to balance. It is the soil from which the framework grew. I hope that as you read my history, you'll begin to see echoes of your own—and realize that wholeness often starts in the places we once felt most broken.

Chapter 1 — Before the Beginning: The Ache for Wholeness

I was raised in a backwoods version of Pentecostal Holiness where salvation came with a dress code. Women wore only long skirts, never cut their hair, and faced suspicion for a dab of makeup, nail polish, or a pair of earrings. Holiness was measured in inches and silence. As a child, I wanted nothing more than to belong, yet every rule seemed to set me further apart from the other children at school.

We moved through churches like tumbleweeds—welcomed, tested, then quietly pushed out when tensions arose. By the time I reached adolescence, I had learned two lessons: community could vanish overnight, and my body was something to hide and be ashamed of.

My mother's skin carried the bronze of her Native American ancestry, a beauty she covered under long sleeves and wide-brimmed hats, like her mother before her, because she had been taught to feel ashamed of it. Watching her hide from the sun was my first lesson in body rejection.

The second came from my siblings, particularly my older brother, who was the most cruel. Their teasing turned the dinner table into a daily trial. *"Four-by-four can't fit through the kitchen door,"* they'd all laugh, my parents included. Or *"four eyes,"* or *"bulldog nose."* It sounds small now, but to a child, those words carried the heavy weight of truth and the heavier weight of rejection.

In the place I should have felt safest, wrapped in belonging, I learned instead what it meant to feel exposed and unprotected—a home that echoed more with ridicule than refuge. The walls that held my laughter also held my deepest wounds. Home should have been my sanctuary, but instead, it became the first battlefield where I learned to armor my heart. I began to see myself not as a person, but as a problem to be fixed.

Diet culture was the air we breathed. My mother cycled through every new promise of thinness—from the grapefruit diet to the cabbage soup diet, from chocolate appetite suppressants called Ayds to over-the-counter diet pills. I watched Mom struggle with self-hatred and low self-esteem.

By five, I had already learned the secret comfort of food. I remember overeating to the point of vomiting more than once. When I was twelve, the family doctor put me on the infamous tuna-fish-only diet: breakfast, lunch, and dinner from a can. I was twelve years old and was already being trained to distrust my hunger. No one taught me what real nourishment meant; they only taught me to wage war against my body. By adulthood, that comfort had hardened into a binge-eating disorder, low self-esteem, and a belief that my value depended on the scale.

The 1990s blurred into survival. I learned to excel in school but faltered everywhere else. College opened a crack of light—psychology courses that whispered new truths about the mind and behavior. (Here's a little secret few people tell: I majored in psychology because I wanted to fix myself. That is an all-too-common story. Now you know.) Psychology gave language to things I had felt but never named: shame, self-efficacy, trauma. I began to see that my eating disorder wasn't gluttony or lack of discipline; it was an attempt to self-soothe in a world that never felt safe.

Still, theory is easier than applying the knowledge in a practical way so that healing can begin. I married and divorced. Twice. I stumbled into relationships that mirrored my wounds, and endured the cycle of abuse that tells you suffering is normal. Each heartbreak added another layer to my armor.

The one bright spot came in 2013, when I met my husband, Todd. Through his steadiness and kindness, I experienced safety for the first time in my life. As that safety took root, my body began to heal. The illnesses that had plagued me for more than two decades slowly disappeared, and for the first time, I found myself moving toward both a healthy body and a peaceful mind.

My husband, Todd, joined me, and together we began cleaning out our pantry and our habits. We quit smoking and drinking, legalized our marriage covenant, and turned repentance into a lifestyle. For the first time, our choices began to align with our prayers.

We tried everything, then settled on low-carb, keto. It was all the rage, and everyone was raving about. The problem is, I only felt better for a short time, all the while, my labs still stayed well within the danger zone.

My body forced the reckoning. Type II diabetes, high blood pressure, fatty liver, kidney damage—my medical chart read like a cautionary tale. By my early forties, I was taking eight prescriptions a day. When eczema erupted over ninety percent of my body, the dermatologist handed me steroids that only worsened everything else. I remember sitting on the edge of my bed, crying because the itching and burning were so fierce I could barely sleep, praying for a reason to keep trying. The thought came as clear as breath: *If you don't change, you will die—and not just physically.*

After going to an allergist and getting no answers again, I started researching like I was back in college. I learned about the elimination diet. That was not an easy feat, but I finally found out what was causing the horrendous eczema that was causing, in addition to the itching, severe nerve pain that even affected my fingernail beds: dairy and peppers.

Another piece of the puzzle fell into place. So, I started studying the relationship between health and diets, and ran across the Blue Zones and the work of Dr Colin Campbell in *The China Study*. After listening to lecture after lecture from one plant-based doctor to another, and reading everything I could get my hands on about diet and health, Todd and I came to the obvious conclusion that if we wanted to feel better and live a longer, healthier life, we had to change *everything*!

Then came the anger. Why had no doctor told me diabetes could be reversed? Why had I been taught to fear food but never taught to love my body? The fury could have consumed me, but instead, it became fuel.

I started writing to process the journey, launching *Healthy in Heart* as a space to research, question, and share. The articles mixed psychology, faith, and wellness long before I knew they were forming the foundation of RISE. Readers began to respond, saying the words permitted them to hope again. Hope is contagious.

That was 2014, the year I stopped handing over my health to others. I began reading every credible study I could find, searching for the cause instead of suppressing the symptoms. I shifted my trust from the medical system to the Creator, who designed all the body's systems. Fasting and prayer led me to small revelations: that food could heal, that emotions could speak through symptoms, and that faith and physiology were not enemies.

Then in 2019, my youngest sister, Pamela, died under horrific circumstances, and my health was also shattered. Grief pulled the floor from beneath me; weight returned, faith cracked, and all the tidy doctrines of my childhood proved too small to hold the pain. Yet even then, something in me refused to die. I sensed that beneath the rubble of religion, diet, and shame, a deeper wholeness was waiting.

Through it all ran a single longing—not merely to be healthy, but to be whole. Wholeness meant harmony between belief and biology, between body and spirit, between what I said I valued and how I actually lived those values.

It meant forgiving my younger self for every binge, every diet, every desperate attempt to be enough. It meant seeing my story not as failure but as fertile ground.

My thoughts, my stress, my sleep, my pace—all of it contributed to either health or dis-ease. The revelation was simple, but life-changing:

Everything affects everything.

That sentence became the cornerstone of my philosophy.

Looking back now, I can trace the thread: a childhood that taught me shame, a lifetime that taught me compassion, an illness that taught me agency. Every pain became purpose, every imbalance a teacher. When people ask where RISE came from, I tell them it started in those long nights of itching and praying, when I realized the body doesn't lie. It tells the truth we're too afraid to speak out loud. And if we listen long enough, it leads us home.

Reflection Prompt

What longing in your life has always been calling you toward balance?

Write freely—without judgment—about the part of you that has never stopped searching for wholeness. That voice is not a weakness; it's your compass.

Chapter 2 — When the Student Is Ready, A Teacher Appears

I have learned that guidance rarely arrives when we feel prepared; it shows up when we are desperate enough to listen. After years of chasing health through every quick fix, I had reached the point where I finally stopped pretending that I could fix myself by willpower alone. I was sick, frightened, and—most importantly—teachable. That was the season when Karen appeared.

Meeting Karen

Karen Smith didn't come wrapped in credentials, though she did have them, and she didn't come in a white coat. When I first met her, she was the registered dietitian at Barnard Medical Center. Her approach was unlike any dietitian I had seen in the past. She came with a curiosity, a calmness, and the kind of listening that made me feel seen rather than studied. Her voice carried the patience of someone who had wrestled with her own shadows and come out gentler on the other side. Where doctors had given me prescriptions, she handed me questions. "What is your body trying to say?" she would ask. No one had ever asked me that before.

Under her tutorship, healing stopped being a linear project and became a dialogue—a relationship between my body, my mind, and something deeper that I can only call spirit. Karen taught me to watch, to document, to run little experiments on myself: change one variable, observe, record, learn. She taught me that data is holy when it's used to serve awareness.

The First Experiments

At first, I treated her advice like homework. I kept notebooks of meals, moods, and sleep. (I still write down all of my meals, even if it is in abbreviated form now.) Patterns began to emerge—the way anxiety bloomed after processed foods or how calm returned after a walk outside. I discovered that sugar wasn't only inflaming my body; it was muting my intuition. Caffeine sharpened focus but stole gentleness and played havoc with my blood sugar. Each discovery made me less afraid of my symptoms and more interested in their meaning.

Karen never dictated a single diet plan. She got me to thinking about my body as my laboratory. So, I learned to "Run the test," while remembering that I am both the scientist and the subject. That approach freed me from the tyranny of perfection. I didn't have to follow anyone else's blueprint; I could co-create one with my Creator. For the first time, I began to respect the intelligence of my own cells.

She also taught me belief acceptance—the radical act of meeting myself where I was rather than fighting what was. I realized that healing doesn't start when I hate my current condition; it started when I finally make peace with reality long enough to learn from it. The moment I stopped waging war on my body, I began to hear its wisdom.

Remembering the Roots

Karen's lessons resonated because they sounded strangely familiar. Long before I knew the word holistic, my grandmother and mother had lived it in quiet ways. Both carried our Native American ancestry with a reverence for the land. They taught me never to take all that a plant offered—always leave some for regeneration, always use the whole of what you harvest. I remember watching my grandmother crush leaves between her palms and breathe in their scent as if greeting an old friend. She would whisper stories about plants that soothed fevers or calmed nerves. "The earth will teach you," she'd say, "if you don't talk over it."

Those early teachings slept inside me for years until Karen awakened them. Karen reframed the same principles in modern language: sustainability, reciprocity, respect for systems. The Cherokee wisdom of using the whole plant mirrored the holistic truth that you cannot separate a person's parts and still call them whole. Where my grandmother brewed teas, Karen brewed awareness. Both women honored the circle of life—nothing wasted, nothing taken without gratitude.

New Voices, New Sciences

As my curiosity widened, new mentors joined the circle—teachers I met through screens and pages rather than face-to-face. Dr. John Bergman was one of the first. His lectures introduced me to the hidden world of toxins: the chemicals in our shampoos, the plastics that leach into our food, the perfumes that disrupt hormones, the neurotoxicity of fluorine that is put into water. He insisted that we are not a collection of replaceable parts, but an integrated being whose systems sing in harmony or discord, depending on how we treat them. "Every cell is listening." That sentence stuck with me—in a good way.

Then came Dr. John McDougall, Dr. Caldwell Esselstyn, Dr. T. Colin Campbell, and Dr. Neal Barnard, along with several physicians at the Barnard Medical Center. From them, I learned that food is not neutral; it is information for the cells. They demonstrated, with data and compassion, that a plant-based diet can reverse disease, unclog arteries, stabilize blood sugar, and literally rewrite cellular memory. I began to see produce aisles as pharmacies designed by GOD Himself.

Dr. Doug Lyle's work on the biology of food addiction cracked open another piece of my puzzle. For decades, I had blamed my lack of willpower; he showed me it was biology doing its best to survive in a world engineered to exploit cravings. His work turned shame into a strategy. Once I understood that dopamine hijacks could be healed rather than condemned, I got the first taste of freedom.

And then there was Dr. Alan Goldhammer, whose studies on water-only fasting revealed the body's innate desire to heal when given the right conditions. He used a simple metaphor that changed everything: if you hit your hand with a hammer every day, the first step to healing isn't medicine—**it's to stop hitting your hand**. I saw myself clearly then: all my "hammers" of processed foods, self-criticism, and overwork. Removing them was not deprivation; it was mercy.

Faith and Inquiry

Amid the studies, another voice entered—Ross K. Nichols. Ross taught through Scripture, history, the humility of unlearning, and the importance of being honest with the text. His teachings reminded me that faith is strongest when it welcomes questions. Truth doesn't fear examination.

His teachings freed me from the dogma of either-or thinking, and I began to realize that more than one thing can be true at the same time. I began to approach wellness in a similar way—no longer choosing between medicine and prayer, research and revelation. Integration became my compass.

Ross's method of study felt like an echo of my own journey. He encouraged digging beneath tradition, searching context, holding tension without fear. That permission changed everything. It allowed me to pursue spirituality as exploration rather than obligation. It also laid the intellectual groundwork for what would later become the Intentional anchor of RISE™—choosing clarity over conformity.

A Whole Being, Not Parts

As these teachers overlapped—Karen's intuition, my grandmother's earth wisdom, the physicians' data, and Ross's theology—a single theme kept surfacing: we are whole. Every aspect of life is interconnected with every other. My emotional wounds shaped my appetite; my food choices influenced my mood; my beliefs affected my biology. Western medicine had taught me to treat systems as separate; my new mentors revealed they were never meant to be divided.

I began teaching myself a new literacy: listening. Instead of labeling symptoms as enemies, I asked what they were trying to communicate. Fatigue may indicate a nutrient deficiency or unspoken grief. Headaches could come from dehydration or from holding in too many "yeses" that should have been "no." Each signal invited partnership rather than punishment.

The Turning Point: Embodiment

Knowledge came easy to me; embodiment did not. For years, I had been collecting facts the way others collect souvenirs—proof that I had visited healing, not that I lived there. I could cite studies on insulin resistance while ignoring the stress that spiked my own glucose levels. Information without embodiment left my soul starving. My husband noticed. One afternoon he looked me in the eye and said, "You don't need another book. You need to breathe."

So, we started simple. Breathing before eating. Blessing water before drinking. Walking barefoot on the grass to remind my nervous system that safety still existed. These small acts built bridges between brain and body. I discovered that peace was not a theory; it was a physiological state I could cultivate. My body, once the enemy, became an ally.

Experiment as Prayer

Running experiments became a form of devotion. Each week, I'd pick one focus—sleep earlier, meditate, eat more greens, or reduce caffeine—and treat the process like a combination of research and prayer. When something worked, gratitude reinforced it; when it didn't, curiosity replaced guilt. The data became personal scripture that was written in heartbeats and hormone levels. Over time, I noticed that failure only happened when I tried to mimic someone else's rhythm. Success came when I listened inwardly. Balance wasn't external; it was attunement.

Bridging Science and Spirit

The more I studied biology, the more it mirrored theology. The body renews itself daily; the soul calls that grace. Cells die and resurrect; Scripture calls that restoration. Circadian rhythms echo Sabbath rhythms—work and rest in divine cadence. It struck me that creation had been preaching wellness since the beginning; however, we forgot how to interpret the sermon.

My mentors had given me vocabulary for every layer. Each contributed a piece of what would become the fourfold framework of RISE. From Karen came Rooted—grounded awareness. From Ross, Intentional—thoughtful discernment. From my medical mentors, Strong—evidence-based resilience. From my grandmother and Goldhammer alike, Energized—life aligned with natural design.

Healing as Humility

The deeper I went, the more I realized that healing wasn't an achievement; it was a matter of humility. It required admitting that the body often knows before the brain does, that intuition is a form of intelligence, and that the Creator encoded guidance into every living system. I learned to stop demanding instant results and start honoring the process. Healing became a conversation between what was wounded and what was wise within me.

Integrating the Lessons

By 2020, the mosaic of influences had fused into a coherent worldview. I no longer saw Karen's gentle questioning and peer-reviewed research as opposites. They were complementary languages pointing toward the same truth: the body is designed for balance. When I finally accepted that, something within me settled. The war ended. From that acknowledgement, peace and creativity bloomed. Articles, teachings, and the early drafts of what would become the RISE framework began to pour out.

I understood then that every teacher had appeared exactly when I was ready for their lesson—and that some disappeared when I was ready to embody the lesson myself.

Balance isn't something you find; it's something you keep creating. The inner ecosystem, a landscape of nerves, hormones, and emotions, requires tending just as surely as a garden does. Stress is drought, while kindness is rainfall.

Every thought releases chemistry.

Every feeling has a physical echo.

Reflection Prompt

Who first modeled the kind of balance you now seek to live?

Think of a person—living or gone—whose way of being radiates steadiness. What qualities do they carry that your soul recognizes as home? How might you begin to cultivate those same qualities in yourself today?

Chapter 3 — From Student to Seeker: The Healing Journey Unfolds

There comes a moment in every apprenticeship when the notes no longer suffice. You can quote the wisdom, trace the diagrams, repeat the steps, but something inside whispers: *Now live it.* That whisper became the soundtrack of my next season. Karen was not a mentor in the traditional sense, but through our weekly class that later grew into the RISE Momentum Circle, I encountered ideas that reshaped how I understood my body and my health. Around me were the voices of physicians, researchers, and spiritual teachers, filling my shelves with insight. Yet knowledge is a lantern, not a destination. It only matters if you're willing to carry it —it only lights the path if you're willing to walk.

When Lessons Leave the Classroom

My classroom became my kitchen, my emotions, my calendar, my journal. Every choice was an experiment. I replaced processed snacks with vegetables, then watched old cravings roar like offended dragons. I adjusted my sleep and felt my moods shift within days. I journaled every reaction—not as judgment, but as conversation. Some days I passed the test; other days I crumpled into exhaustion and began again. Healing, I discovered, is cyclical, not linear. You continue to circle the same lessons until they imprint on your muscle memory.

The body does not lie, but it also does not rush. I learned this the hard way each time I expected instant results. When my blood sugar spiked after a stressful day, I wanted to blame food. I began to look deeper—not only at what I ate, but at everything I was allowing to shape me. I started looking deeper, and I began asking myself: "What else did I consume today?"

Often it wasn't sugar; it was fear, hurry, or resentment. Slowly, I began to translate physical symptoms into emotional language. A tension headache might mean I'd swallowed too many unspoken words. Bloating can point to something unprocessed in the spirit as much as in the digestive system —because the mind and body are never as separate as we imagine.

Living the lessons meant surrendering my old identity as the good student—the one who performed well to earn approval. I had to learn self-trust more than self-control. That shift felt like a toddler walking for the first time without holding on to the couch: exhilarating and terrifying in equal measure.

The Body as Teacher

During that period, my health swung like a pendulum. Some weeks I felt radiant; others I could barely climb stairs. Each swing exposed another layer of imbalance. My body, once an enemy and later an experiment, became my tutor. It told me when I was grounded

(Rooted) and when I was drifting. It warned me when habits were mechanical rather than mindful (Intentional). It tested my resilience through flare-ups that demanded perseverance (Strong). And in rare, luminous moments, it rewarded me with vitality so pure it felt holy (Energized).

Those four words—Rooted, Intentional, Strong, Energized—didn't arrive all at once. They surfaced gradually, like stones emerging as the tide receded. I noticed I wrote them often in my journal margins, sometimes capitalized, sometimes circled. They became signposts marking my growth:

- ○ Rooted when I stayed present instead of escaping into old numbing patterns.
- ○ Intentional when my choices aligned with my values.
- ○ Strong when I held boundaries or showed up despite fear.
- ○ Energized when peace replaced fatigue because body, mind, and spirit were finally in rhythm.

At first, I treated them as adjectives; eventually, I realized they described a framework taking shape inside me.

Experiment, Fail, Adjust, Repeat

Living holistically sounds graceful in theory.

In practice, though, it is quite messy.

There were nights when grief still drove me to the pantry. Days when stress silenced prayer. Times when the perfectionist in me tallied every "failure" as proof that I was unworthy of teaching others. But each stumble became data. The scientist in me noted triggers; the seeker in me asked for grace.

I discovered that transformation doesn't demand constant success—it requires continuous return. Every relapse into old habits was an invitation to start the cycle again, this time with more awareness. I began to measure progress not by how few mistakes I made but by how quickly I came back after making them. Recovery, I realized, isn't about perfection; it's about shortening the distance between falling and rising.

The Illusion of Perfection

Perfectionism had been my longest addiction. It masqueraded as discipline but was rooted in fear—fear of judgment, rejection, failure. Growing up, approval was conditional; belonging was fragile. My grades, weight, and spiritual performance became currency for love. That mindset bled into adulthood. Every health plan I followed became another religion of rules. Miss a step, and shame came roaring back.

Psychology refers to this as conditional self-worth, which corrodes both self-esteem and self-efficacy. When your worth depends on flawless performance, even success feels temporary. You live in perpetual vigilance, waiting for the next mistake to prove you unworthy again.

It's exhausting.

My nervous system lived in fight-or-flight even when nothing was chasing me. My blood pressure numbers rose in agreement.

Breaking that cycle required something radical: compassion. Not the Hallmark version, but the gritty kind that faces imperfection and stays. I began to practice talking to myself the way I would to a frightened child. When I binged, instead of "You failed again," I whispered, "You must be hurting—what do you need?" At first, it felt fake, even weak. Then I noticed my binge episodes shrinking, my recovery time shortening. Compassion wasn't indulgence; it was medicine.

Moments of Breakdown and Breakthrough

One winter morning, exhaustion hit so hard that I sat on the kitchen floor and cried among the groceries. The scale hadn't moved in months, my labs stalled, and I feared I was fooling myself. Then I noticed the sunlight spilling across the floor—warm, steady, indifferent to my meltdown. In that moment, I sensed the gentle truth: You are not failing; you are unfolding.

My body had carried me through every binge, every heartbreak, every sleepless night, and every storm I thought I wouldn't survive. Even when I numbed it, ignored its signals, or spoke to it like an enemy, it still showed up for me—heart beating faithfully, breathing steady, and believing I might one day come home to it. I began to see that my body had never betrayed me; I had betrayed its trust.

Healing takes time because trust takes time. My body needed to trust that I wouldn't abandon it again.

From that day, I shifted my prayers from "Make me well" to "Teach me how to live well." That change of language changed everything. It turned desperation into dialogue. Instead of begging for rescue, I began collaborating with grace.

Breakthroughs followed in unexpected places: in the quiet rhythm of chopping vegetables, in the steadiness of daily walks, in laughter shared with Todd and Kelsey. Joy began to return—not the ecstatic high of accomplishment, but the soft joy of consistency. Peace became palpable — something you could feel straight through to the soul.

Becoming Rooted

Rootedness, I learned, isn't stillness; it's stability. A tree sways because it is flexible, not because it is weak. My roots deepened through routine: morning journaling, Scripture or reflection, herbal tea, ten minutes of silence before screens, and weekly meal planning. These rituals weren't rules; they were reminders. They tethered me to the present moment. Whenever anxiety pulled me into future catastrophes, I asked, "Where are my feet?" That question grounded me faster than any medication ever could.

My Native heritage resurfaced here, too. I started gardening again, touching the soil, remembering the elders' teaching that every plant carries a lesson. Weeds taught persistence, flowers taught generosity, seasons taught surrender. The earth became both a metaphor and a mirror for my internal growth.

Practicing Intention

Intentional living meant making choices aligned with my deepest yes. It required pausing before autopilot. Do I actually want this food, this conversation, this schedule? That slight pause rewired my nervous system. It introduced agency where habit once ruled. Over time, intention replaced impulse.

I learned to use intention even in rest. Instead of collapsing into Netflix guilt, I chose to rest consciously—lighting a candle, breathing, acknowledging the sacredness of restoration. Intention transformed ordinary acts into spiritual practice. Washing dishes became a gift of gratitude; folding laundry became a form of prayer.

Discovering Strength

Strength had always looked like pushing harder, lifting heavier, enduring longer. But the kind of strength that sustains wellness is quieter. It's the ability to say no, to rest, to ask for help. I learned that discipline divorced from compassion becomes punishment. True strength integrates both boundaries and grace.

When setbacks came—a flare of eczema, an emotional trigger—I practiced holding my ground internally. Instead of collapsing into self-blame, I reminded myself that I am still in process. Strength became trust during the process. It wasn't the absence of weakness; it was the refusal to interpret weakness as failure.

Awakening Energy

Energy was the by-product of alignment. As I ate cleaner foods, slept in sync with the sun, and reduced chemical exposures, my vitality returned. But the deeper energy came from purpose. Teaching small groups, sharing articles, writing books, and mentoring others reignited something deep in my spirit.

Service produced a current that caffeine never could. I realized energy flows wherever love is not blocked. When resentment built up, my energy stalled; when gratitude flowed, strength followed.

Lifestyle Experiments That Worked—and Didn't

Some experiments became lifelong habits:

- o Morning light exposure within an hour of waking balanced my circadian rhythm.
- o Intermittent fasting restored insulin sensitivity.

- Whole-food plant-based, low-fat, no added sugar eating lowered my inflammation markers.
- Journaling emotions before meals reduced binge triggers.

Others didn't stick. Extreme detoxes backfired; over-exercise spiked stress hormones. Each failure refined discernment. The goal wasn't to master everything; it was to understand myself.

I also learned the value of community accountability. Sharing progress with friends kept me honest and connected. Isolation breeds relapse; belonging breeds resilience. When people joined me in experimenting with recipes or gratitude lists, healing multiplied, and that communal rhythm became the seed for what would later evolve into the 9 Pillars of RISE (these will be covered in a future book, a brief overview is included in Appendix E).

The Psychology of Self-Compassion

My psychology background gave me vocabulary for what my spirit already knew. Research by Dr. Kristin Neff defines self-compassion through three components: self-kindness, common humanity, and mindfulness. Applying them daily changed my internal dialogue.

- Self-kindness: speaking to myself as I would to someone I love.
- Common humanity: remembering everyone struggles; imperfection connects us.
- Mindfulness: observing pain without fusing with it.

These practices rewired the negative self-talk patterns that had been forged in childhood shame. Each compassionate thought calmed my amygdala, reduced cortisol levels, and created space for my healing biology to do its work. Science validated what faith had always taught: love casts out fear—even at the cellular level.

Integrating Mind, Body, and Spirit

By this stage, the line between disciplines disappeared. Science explained mechanisms; spirituality gave them meaning. Prayer influenced parasympathetic tone; gratitude shifted neurotransmitters; forgiveness lowered blood pressure. The Creator had woven physiology and faith into the same tapestry.

I began mapping my healing like concentric circles:

1. Physical – nutrition, movement, rest.

2. Emotional – self-regulation, healthy boundaries.

3. Mental – thought renewal, learning.

4. Spiritual – connection, surrender, purpose.

When all four circles overlapped, I felt harmony—a living preview of what I would later call "the circle of wholeness." It wasn't constant, but it was attainable.

Facing Relapse Without Regression

Life has continued to test me. During stressful seasons—family illness, someone trying to damage my reputation, sibling rejection, workload spikes—the old coping patterns whispered. But now I recognize them sooner. I treat relapse as feedback, not failure. Each time, I recover faster. Neuroplasticity is on my side; every repetition of self-compassion strengthens new neural pathways.

The most incredible freedom came when I realized I didn't have to earn healing. I only had to cooperate with it. My body wanted balance as much as my soul did. My job was to stop interrupting the process with shame and resistance.

The Shift from Student to Seeker

Somewhere in the midst of experiments and articles, I stopped asking, "Who or what will fix me?" and started asking, "What can I learn from this?"

That was the day the student became the seeker. Seeking is different from striving. Striving chases outcomes; whereas seeking treasures the wisdom gained along the journey. The seeker understands that arrival is an illusion—every revelation gives birth to new curiosity.

This posture of seeking kept me humble and hungry. It prevented me from turning new knowledge into new dogma. I remained open and teachable, yet discerning. The humility of seeking birthed the first whispers of mentorship in me; I wanted to help others discover their own experiments of grace.

Defining the Four Emerging Themes

By the end of this chapter of my life, the four RISE anchors stood clear:

1. Rooted in Truth – Stability grows from honesty. Healing requires acknowledging what is, not fantasizing about what could, would, or should be.
2. Intentional in Habit – Small consistent choices sculpt destiny more than any grand declarations.
3. Strong in Spirit – Resilience is spiritual stamina—the ability to bend but not break.
4. Energized for Hope – Hope itself generates energy; when we believe renewal is possible, physiology follows.

These weren't slogans; they were coordinates for navigation. Whenever I lost direction, I asked which of the four had drifted. The answer always revealed the next step.

Learning to Rest Inside the Process

One of the final lessons of this phase was rest—not as a reward, but as a rhythm. I began observing the weekly Sabbath commanded in the Ten Commandments: a deliberate ceasing, one set-apart day each week. It wasn't escapism or self-care dressed up in spiritual language. It was obedience that required trust—trust in God, and trust in the way the body was designed to recover.

And you know what? The world didn't collapse when I stopped. My body actually thanked me. Energy in the following week felt fundamentally different after a genuine Sabbath, after ceasing from Friday night to Saturday night. Science calls it circaseptan recovery. I came to recognize it as grace, embedded in the Creator's wisdom long before we learned how to measure it.

Emerging from the Cocoon

Looking back, the transformation was subtle but undeniable. I hadn't become someone new; I had finally met the person I'd always been beneath layers of coping. I felt lighter, not just in pounds but in presence. The mirror no longer frightened me. I could see a woman in progress rather than a problem to solve.

The student in me still studies; the seeker in me now leads. Every lesson I teach through RISE—every journal prompt, every group discussion—traces its lineage to this messy middle where I learned to live what I once merely believed. These pages are not about perfection; they're about permission: permission to be unfinished, to experiment, to rest, and to rise again.

Reflection Prompt

What lesson keeps returning until you embody it?

Write about a pattern that revisits your life—a theme, challenge, or habit that won't release you until you integrate its wisdom. Notice how the repetition isn't punishment but persistence—the universe's way of ensuring you don't graduate without learning what matters most.

Chapter 4 — Seeds of a Framework: When Life Began to Speak in Patterns

The shift from healing to teaching didn't happen overnight. It began quietly—ink stains on journal pages, fragments of insight scribbled in the margins of grocery lists, and conversations that refused to leave my mind. Long before the RISE framework had a name, it lived as a pattern whispering through every lesson life gave me.

I began to notice that what worked in one area of life mirrored what worked in another. What healed my body also soothed my mind; what freed my emotions restored my spirit. It was as though creation itself was tutoring me, repeating the same theme until I was ready to hear it: everything is connected, and everything repeats.

And everything affects everything!

Listening for the Echo

Patterns are teachers. They repeat not to punish but to reinforce, like waves carving the shoreline until the shape finally holds. For years, I had mistaken repetition for failure—another diet, another relapse, another heartbreak. But one morning, reading through my old journals, I noticed something different. Each "failure" carried the same core lesson dressed in new circumstances: trust, surrender, consistency, compassion. The same few truths recirculated again and again, patiently awaiting embodiment.

I began to call this the "divine curriculum." When a lesson reappears, it isn't punishment; it's an invitation. My own curriculum wasn't abstract or lofty—it was painfully practical, and it repeated until I finally listened. The same four lessons kept returning in different forms: learning my worth without earning it, setting healthy boundaries without guilt, facing my emotions instead of numbing or spiritualizing them, and stewarding my energy so I wasn't living in constant depletion. Whenever life spun out of balance, one of these had been neglected. Only later did I recognize how naturally these lessons would fit within the RISE framework—not because I imposed a system on my life, but because my life had already been teaching me what Rooted, Intentional, Strong, and Energized living actually requires.

Journals as Data

I had always kept journals, but now they became laboratories. Each entry documented choices, emotions, foods, triggers, and insights. Patterns leapt off the page. When I was grounded—taking walks, praying, eating from the garden—my entries brimmed with peace and gratitude. When I over-scheduled, skipped rest, or ignored boundaries, chaos followed. It didn't matter whether the topic was health, relationships, or finances—the same principle held: what was rooted thrived; what was rushed withered.

Reading months of entries at once felt like watching time-lapse photography of my own soul. I could see cause-and-effect linking like constellations. A bad happening predicted emotional eating; emotional eating predicted guilt; guilt predicted isolation. But when I inserted intention—a plan, a pause, a prayer—the spiral softened. The data didn't lie, and the balance wasn't luck. It was rhythm.

From Private Notes to Shared Stories

As my confidence grew, I began sharing small reflections online through Healthy in Heart. What surprised me most was how universal my "personal" discoveries were. People I'd never met wrote back: "I thought I was the only one who felt that way." Their comments mirrored my own entries almost word-for-word. That was my first glimpse of community as a mirror—the realization that individual healing becomes collective wisdom when spoken aloud.

Soon, readers became friends. We compared notes like researchers of the soul. Each person's story, though unique in detail, followed the same cycle: awareness, resistance, surrender, renewal. It was never linear. We'd move forward three steps, fall back one, pause, and find ourselves changed in subtler ways than before. Healing, we discovered, spirals—it revisits old wounds with a new perspective until integration completes the loop.

Seeing the Geometry of Growth

The more stories I heard, the more visual the pattern became. I started sketching circles, arrows, and overlapping loops in the margins of my notebooks. I noticed that the process of transformation always curved back toward its beginning, but on a higher level—like climbing a spiral staircase. Each turn built upon the last. This geometry felt familiar, almost ancient: seasons, moon phases, circadian rhythm, the very heartbeat pulsing: systole and diastole. Life, it seemed, was a choreography of contraction and expansion.

I drew four quadrants inside the circle and labeled them with the qualities that kept repeating: Rooted, Intentional, Strong, Energized. The order varied depending on context, but the interplay was constant. Grounded truth fed intention; intention then built strength; strength generated energy; energy, when aligned, deepened roots again. The cycle completed itself, a self-sustaining ecosystem of wellness.

At first, I called it "the renewal loop." Later, it would earn its official name: The RISE Circle.

When Life Confirmed the Pattern

By the time friends and readers began resonating with what I was writing, I had years of personal experiments behind me—moments of trial, relapse, revelation, and slow rebuilding. I wasn't teaching anyone; I was telling the truth about what had worked and what hadn't. Yet, as people began sharing their own stories in response, I noticed something: their experiences mirrored my own. The circumstances were different, but the rhythm was the same—awareness, realignment, renewal.

One woman wrote about her constant exhaustion despite "doing everything right." Another person described their battle with emotional eating and the breakthrough that came when they stopped seeing their body as the enemy. Each story reflected one of the four anchors—Rooted, Intentional, Strong, or Energized—and revealed what happens when one area falls out of balance. The pattern I had once doubted began confirming itself through the real lives of my readers.

The more I listened, the clearer it became: this wasn't just my story. It was a shared human rhythm—a framework written into the body, waiting to be remembered.

Cyclical, Not Linear

Culture loves straight lines—progress charts, before-and-after photos, success timelines. But real transformation behaves more like the seasons. Winter is not failure; it's rest disguised as barrenness. The tree that sheds its leaves isn't dying; it's conserving energy for spring. Once I accepted that rhythm, I stopped condemning my pauses. Rest was part of the work.

This revelation dismantled the perfectionism that had haunted me. The old mindset equated consistency with worthiness: if I missed a workout or slipped in my diet, the whole system collapsed. The new paradigm honored return over performance. The question became not "Did I stay perfect?" but "Did I come back?" Healing is fidelity to the process, not obedience to the plan.

I began teaching this principle to others: expect the cycle. When discouragement hits, name the season rather than judging it. If you're in a winter of healing, don't uproot the tree. Trust the pattern—its roots are working underground.

Integrating Science and Spirit

Around this time, my fascination with patterns led me into the science of circadian and ultradian rhythms. I learned how every cell in the body follows daily cycles of light and dark, work and rest. The parallels to spiritual renewal were uncanny.

Morning cortisol rises to awaken us while melatonin rises at night to repair us. Even the immune system, digestive tract, and emotions follow the same ebb and flow. I realized that creation itself testifies to the truth of rhythm. We were designed for balance because balance is built into the Creation.

This discovery deepened my respect for the Creator's design. My earlier mentors had taught me to question tradition; now science confirmed what ancient wisdom already knew: we thrive in cycles, not straight lines. Modern culture's insistence on constant output is biologically impossible and spiritually destructive. The RISE Circle became my personal rebellion against linear living—a return to the divine geometry of renewal.

The Anatomy of the Circle

I refined the sketch until it felt whole. The circle contained four quadrants intersected by a smaller inner ring labeled "Awareness." Awareness was the pivot point connecting them all, because without awareness, no transformation holds.

- **Rooted** — the practice of grounding in truth, values, and belonging.
- **Intentional** — conscious alignment of choices with purpose.
- **Strong** — resilience built through boundaries and perseverance.
- **Energized** — vitality generated through alignment and rest.

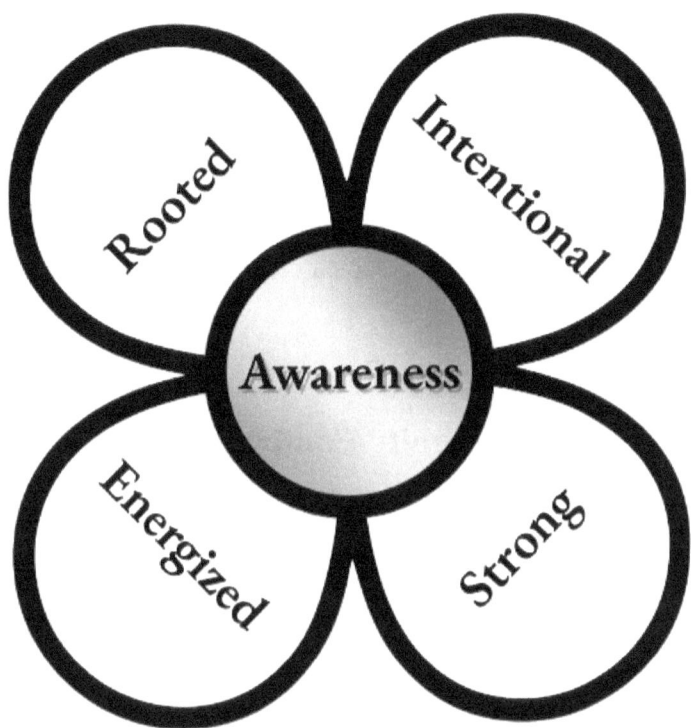

Moving clockwise through the circle created momentum; moving counter-clockwise revealed regression. But even regression had purpose—it showed where to re-enter the flow. I tested this model on myself for months, tracking moods and decisions. The accuracy startled me. When fatigue appeared, the energy quadrant was empty. When anxiety rose, the rooted quadrant became unstable. When procrastination crept in, the intention quadrant blurred. The circle became both a diagnostic tool and a compass.

From Personal Framework to Collective Language

When I began teaching these principles publicly, people responded instantly. They said the circle gave shape to something they had felt but never articulated. It was inclusive enough to fit any belief system yet specific enough to guide daily choices. Christians saw echoes of the fruit of the Spirit; psychologists saw behavioral cycles; scientists saw feedback loops. The framework didn't argue with any worldview—it harmonized them.

This universality convinced me that RISE wasn't just mine. It belonged to anyone ready to listen to life's patterns. I became less of an inventor and more of a translator, putting words to a rhythm that had always existed.

Community Confirmation

The first time I drew the circle for a small group, silence filled the room. Then one lady whispered, "That's exactly what my year looked like." Another pointed to a quadrant and said, "That's where I got stuck." We spent hours mapping individual stories onto the model—relationships, health journeys, grief recoveries—and every timeline curved into the same circle of return.

These sessions birthed what I called "RISE Mapping." We treated personal stories like weather patterns, tracing where storms formed and where calm returned. The process provided people with a language for progress that isn't linear. Someone who felt "back at square one" realized they were actually on the next rotation of the spiral, revisiting the same lesson with new wisdom. The relief in their faces confirmed what I already knew: hope grows where patterns make sense.

Patterns in Creation

Outside of our meeting rooms, creation continued to preach the same sermon. The moon waxed and waned; tides advanced and retreated; seeds broke open only in darkness. Even breath itself follows a circle—inhalation, pause, exhalation, pause. The more I noticed, the more impossible it became to separate physical law from spiritual metaphor. Everything lived and healed through rhythm.

I began structuring my life accordingly. Work followed daylight; rest followed sunset. I planned creative seasons and reflective seasons, growth cycles and pruning cycles. Productivity rose, but more importantly, peace returned. The circle was no longer theory—it was a lived theology.

Naming the Framework

The acronym RISE arrived one morning during prayer and journaling. I had been meditating on themes of restoration—the idea that we fall only to rise higher. The words Rooted, Intentional, Strong, Energized appeared almost simultaneously. They captured both the vertical motion of growth and the cyclical motion of rhythm. To rise is not to escape the ground but to draw nourishment from it.

Naming the framework felt like naming a child: the essence was already there; I merely recognized it. I traced the letters in my notebook and felt the quiet confirmation that this was the language through which I would serve others.

The Philosophy Crystallizes

As I integrated years of data, dialogue, and reflection, the philosophy behind RISE crystallized:

1. Healing is relational. Mind, body, and spirit communicate constantly; wellness depends on keeping that conversation honest.

2. Growth is rhythmic. Progress repeats in spirals; relapse is part of refinement.
3. Truth is inclusive. Science and spirituality are not rivals, but reflections of each other.
4. Balance is dynamic. Wholeness adapts with the seasons, never remaining static.

These truths became the backbone of every future RISE book, course, and journal. But at this stage, they lived simply as awe. I would sit at my desk, pen hovering, marveling that decades of pain had arranged themselves into order.

The chaos had coherence after all.

Lessons from the Pattern

The more I studied these patterns, the more they taught me humility. Life repeats lessons because love refuses to give up. The same theme will return, wearing new clothes, until we embody it fully. My recurring lessons—trust, rest, self-compassion—were not failures but acts of faithfulness. Each repetition sanded the rough edges of pride and fear, shaping me into someone capable of teaching others gently.

The Call to Share

By the time I officially began writing *RISE*^{TM}*: The Beginning of Balance*, the framework was no longer a concept but a lived reality. Community stories, scientific studies, and spiritual insights all converged into a single message: balance is possible when we cooperate with rhythm. I felt an undeniable call to share—not as an expert, but as a witness. I wanted readers to see their own patterns, to realize that repetition might be grace in disguise.

The act of writing became a sacred pattern itself: inhale inspiration, exhale words, pause, revise, rest. Even the creative process followed the cycle.

Living the Cycle

From this revelation grew the idea for a series of guided journals that would move in harmony with the rhythm of creation. Healing and growth aren't one-time events; they are seasonal returns— spirals, not straight lines. Each journal in the *RISE™ Circle of Wholeness Collection* is designed to span three months, the length of a season, walking through the same circular framework that began as a simple sketch: Rooted, Intentional, Strong, Energized.

Over the course of seven years, these twenty-eight journals form a living cycle—a complete rhythm of renewal that mirrors the turning of the seasons and the lessons they carry. Balance isn't built overnight; it takes time, *awareness*, and repeated practice to grow deep roots and lasting change. Each rotation through the cycle strengthens the next, turning intention into embodiment.

Each year centers on one layer of the circle's wisdom while revisiting the others, creating a rhythm of reflection and reawakening. Spring invites new roots and beginnings. Summer nurtures strength and growth. Autumn calls for intentional harvest and alignment. Winter teaches stillness and restoration. Then, the cycle begins again—deeper, steadier, wiser.

This ongoing rhythm isn't about chasing change but about becoming balanced—learning to rise with each return. You can learn more about these journals at the back of the book in the section titled: Appendix F: The Seven-Year RISE Journey.

Reflection Prompt

What patterns in your own growth keep repeating for a reason?

Review old journals, memories, or seasons of your life. Notice which themes reappear—trust, patience, self-worth, boundaries, surrender, something else entirely? Ask what unfinished lesson those repetitions might be trying to teach. Rather than fighting the recurrence, honor it as the rhythm of your becoming.

Chapter 5 — Staying Upright: Learning Balance From a Tightrope Walker

I once stood in a crowd watching a tightrope walker move slowly across a thin line suspended high above the ground. There was no music swelling, no dramatic buildup. Just a person placing one foot in front of the other, arms slightly extended, eyes forward. The silence was thick with attention.

What struck me was not the height or the danger, but the movement.

She was never still.

At first glance, it looked like balance — calm, controlled, impressive. But the longer I watched, the more I noticed something else entirely. Every step included a correction. A shift of weight. A subtle tilt of the hips. A slight movement of the arms responding to wind, fatigue, or the natural sway of the line beneath her.

Balance was not something she achieved and then held.

Balance was something she responded into, moment by moment.

If she had frozen in place, trying to lock herself into a perfect position, she would have fallen. Staying upright required motion. Awareness. Adjustment. A willingness to respond rather than resist.

That image stayed with me because it quietly contradicted everything I had been taught about balance.

Stability Versus Adjustment

For a long time, I believed balance meant stability without movement. I thought it was something you reached after enough effort, discipline, or self-control. If I could just organize my life correctly, make better choices, or push myself a little harder, balance would finally arrive and stay. I thought that once I reached it, I was done.

But here's the truth: Real life never works that way.

No matter how much I refined my systems or improved my habits, imbalance still showed up. Fatigue. Emotional overload. Overcommitment. A sense of being slightly off-center without being able to explain why. When that happened, I treated it like a personal failure, something I should have anticipated or prevented.

I didn't yet understand that the imbalance wasn't the problem.

My relationship to it was.

Watching the tightrope walker helped me see what I had been missing. Balance is not the absence of sway. It is the ability to notice sway early and respond with accuracy rather than panic.

A tightrope walker does not judge themselves for wobbling. They don't interpret movement as a sign of weakness. Wobble is expected. It is information. The moment they feel it, they adjust — not dramatically, not forcefully, but just enough to bring themselves back into alignment.

They do not overcorrect.

They do not rush.

They do not stop walking to analyze the meaning of the wobble.

They respond.

That is what keeps them upright.

Balance Taught Through Movement

As I watched, I realized this wasn't the first time I had seen balance taught through movement.

When we were girls, my mom used to have us practice walking with a heavy book balanced on our heads. It was part posture lesson, part game, part quiet discipline disguised as play. We would line up, place the book carefully, and start walking across the room, trying our best to keep it steady.

At first, it felt almost impossible. Every step sent the book sliding. Our shoulders tensed. Our necks stiffened. We tried to hold ourselves rigid, convinced that stillness would keep the book in place. It didn't.

What worked instead was awareness. Small adjustments. A subtle shift in how we held our bodies. A softer step. A quieter pace. We learned that balance didn't come from locking ourselves into position. It came from paying attention and responding in time.

There were two very good reasons to pay attention.

The first was the satisfaction of accomplishment. There was something quietly rewarding about making it across the room with the book still balanced. It wasn't about praise or perfection. It was about realizing you could sense what was needed and respond before things went wrong.

The second reason was much more practical. If you didn't notice the shift early — if you waited too long to adjust — the book didn't just fall. It dropped. And when it dropped, it often hit your leg or your foot on the way down.

And that hurt.

What stayed with me wasn't fear of the book falling, but the realization that the pain usually came after ignoring the early signs. The book always warned you first. A tilt. A slide. A change in pressure. If you responded then, the correction was minor and almost effortless. If you didn't, the consequence was sudden and sharp.

We learned, without being told, that noticing sooner mattered.

That lesson lived in my body long before I had language for it.

Early Lesson Reintroduced

Watching the tightrope walker years later, I realized she was doing the same thing. Responding to the earliest signals. Staying attentive rather than rigid. Trusting her ability to adjust instead of fearing imbalance itself.

In my own life, I had been doing the opposite.

When an imbalance appeared, I either ignored it and pushed through or reacted with urgency, trying to fix everything at once. Both responses made the strain worse. I was either enduring without listening or overcorrecting without discernment.

What I hadn't learned yet was how to stay in a relationship with imbalance — to notice it without assigning meaning, and to adjust without turning the adjustment into a judgment about my worth.

The tightrope walker showed me that balance is not something you hold. It is something you inhabit.

She trusted her ability to adjust. That trust changes everything. It allowed her to keep moving without fear, even when conditions changed. Wind picks up. Muscles tire. Focus wavers. None of that signals failure. It simply signals the need for a different response.

Balance Lessons Reapplied

The same is true in a human life.

Energy shifts. Emotions rise. Capacity changes. Seasons demand different things from us. If we expect ourselves to remain perfectly steady through all of it, we end up rigid, anxious, or exhausted. We mistake adaptability for instability and endurance for strength.

But real strength looks more like responsiveness.

The tightrope walker does not grip the line. They don't fight the movement beneath them. They cooperate with it. Their awareness stays wide enough to sense change before it becomes dangerous. Their adjustments are small because they are timely.

That was the lesson I needed.

When I began to apply this way of thinking to my own life, something softened. I stopped waiting until I was overwhelmed to respond. I started paying attention sooner — to the early signs of depletion, tension, or misalignment. A subtle tightening in my chest. A creeping irritability. A sense of being rushed or disconnected.

Those signals weren't accusations. They were feedback.

Instead of asking, "What's wrong with me?" I began asking, "What adjustment would help me stay upright right now?"

Sometimes the answer was simple. Step away. Slow down. Eat. Rest. Say no without explanation. Other times, the adjustment was internal — releasing an expectation, loosening my grip on an outcome, or allowing uncertainty to exist without trying to resolve it immediately.

None of these adjustments fixed my life in a dramatic way. But they restored balance more quickly than any grand declaration ever had.

Other Lessons Learned

I also learned something else from the tightrope walker: balance is maintained while moving. You don't stop living until things feel steady. You learn how to stay attentive while continuing forward. Waiting for perfect conditions is not an option. Balance is dynamic, responsive, and alive.

That realization changed how I understood resilience. Strength was no longer about pushing through discomfort at all costs. It was about staying present enough to adjust before harm occurred. Endurance without awareness is not strength. It is neglect.

Over time, the more I trusted my ability to respond, the less afraid I became of imbalance. I didn't need to control every variable or anticipate every outcome. I could stay upright by listening and adjusting as I went.

This is what the tightrope walker knows in their body.

Balance is not a pose you achieve.

It is a conversation you stay in.

You are not meant to walk your life without sway. You are meant to notice sway early enough to respond with care. When an imbalance appears, it is not a verdict. It is a cue. An invitation to shift your weight, soften your stance, and continue with more awareness than before.

Learning to live this way does not eliminate uncertainty. It builds trust — not in your ability to be perfect, but in your capacity to adjust.

And that trust is what keeps you upright.

Reflection Prompt

Take a moment to reflect, without judgment or urgency:

Where in your life have you been trying to hold balance instead of adjusting into it?

What early signals do you tend to ignore until imbalance becomes unavoidable?

If you trusted your ability to adjust sooner, what small shift might help you stay upright right now?

You don't need to answer everything.

Let the noticing be enough.

Chapter 6 — The Birth of RISE: From Personal Healing to Collective Movement

There are moments in life when everything you've walked through—the pain, the lessons, the loss—suddenly rearranges itself into meaning. You look back and realize none of it was wasted. For me, that realization arrived like fire: fierce, cleansing, impossible to ignore. The ashes of my old life—religious rigidity, body hatred, illness, perfectionism—became the soil where something radiant began to take root. I felt like a phoenix, rising not in triumph but in gratitude. The rising wasn't glamorous; it was sacred. It was the quiet, trembling miracle of being reborn into balance.

From Mantra to Movement

For years, RISE had been my private mantra. I would whisper it during difficult days: Rooted, Intentional, Strong, Energized. The words steadied me when nothing else could. But in 2020, as the world tilted into collective uncertainty, I began to sense that this mantra wasn't meant to remain personal. Friends who followed my health journey kept asking, "What are you doing that's different? How are you staying grounded?" I found myself repeating the same four principles again and again. What had started as my survival code was resonating with others as a blueprint for wholeness.

I began sharing small reflections online, writing posts that wove together psychology, nutrition, spirituality, and self-compassion. The response was immediate. People wrote, "This finally makes sense." They weren't looking for another wellness trend; they were looking for something human—something that honored both science and soul. That was when I realized RISE wasn't just about me getting well; it was about us remembering how to live whole again.

Naming the Anchors

Names have power. Throughout history, naming something has always been an act of creation. As I journaled through the years of healing, four words kept recurring like coordinates on a map. Each one carried its own rhythm, its own truth:

- o Rooted — Stability, truth, belonging, grounding in what is real.
- o Intentional — Conscious choice, clarity, alignment, purpose.
- o Strong — Resilience, boundaries, perseverance through grace.
- o Energized — Vitality, joy, flow, harmony between effort and rest.

Together, they formed a compass. The acronym felt divinely orchestrated: RISE. It captured the motion of healing—not a straight climb, but a continual ascension from ashes to light. To rise is to return to life, again and again.

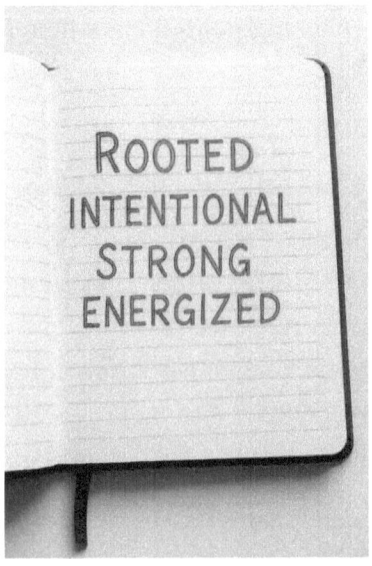

I remember sitting at my desk, tracing the letters in my notebook, and feeling an almost electric recognition. These weren't just nice words; they were the distilled essence of everything I had lived and learned. Each anchor corresponded with one of the four directions, one of the four elements, one of the four aspects of being—body, mind, emotion, and spirit. The symmetry felt ancient and authentic.

The Phoenix Moment

The months leading up to the official naming of RISE were turbulent. I was still managing health flare-ups and processing a world that seemed to be burning. Yet somewhere within the flames, clarity emerged. The phoenix image wouldn't leave me alone. I saw myself—and so many others—standing in the ruins of what no longer served us: toxic diets, broken belief systems, surface-level faith, and cultural noise that called exhaustion "normal." Everything familiar had turned to ash, but the ashes themselves shimmered with possibility.

The legend of the phoenix says that when it burns, it doesn't perish—it purifies. The fire releases what's old so that the essence can return renewed.

That was my story.

I had been through the fires of sickness, shame, and spiritual confusion, but those fires refined me. They burned away the illusion that I needed to be perfect to be whole. They stripped me of dependence on systems that never offered true healing. When I finally emerged, wings singed but intact, I realized: the same flame that destroyed also forged.

RISE became the language of that rebirth. The ashes of religion gave birth to a relationship. The ashes of diet culture metamorphosed into discernment. The ashes of shame yielded way for self-compassion. The ashes of isolation engendered community. I wasn't climbing out of the fire alone anymore—I was reaching back to pull others with me.

The First Sparks of Community

It didn't begin as a plan. The original group had dissolved, and for a while, I thought that was the end of it. But several of us still felt a pull to keep meeting—to stay connected, to keep growing. I reached out to Karen, who had led the previous group, and asked if she knew anyone willing to facilitate a new one. She asked around. I asked around. No one seemed willing—or maybe it just wasn't theirs to carry. Looking back, it felt almost fated.

Finally, I told her, "If no one else will do it, I will." And with that simple yes, Karen handed the torch to me. Karen let everyone know. Not everyone from the original group chose to continue, but those who did formed something new—something deeply rooted in trust and authenticity. From the very beginning, we decided that honesty would be our foundation. I made it my responsibility to go first, to model what openness looks like. When we gather, I share my struggles as freely as my wins, because vulnerability has to start somewhere.

Over time, our RISE Circle evolved into more than just a weekly meeting. It became a refuge—a place where being real matters more than being right. We laugh, cry, and learn together. In the safety of that circle, friendships have taken root, and healing has begun to unfold. What started with a question and a willingness to step forward became the heartbeat of what RISE truly means: showing up, for ourselves and for each other again and again, until balance feels like home.

Belief Acceptance: The Core Difference

From the beginning, I knew RISE had to be different from mainstream wellness programs. Most models operate from a foundation of fixing—fixing the body, fixing the mindset, fixing the flaws. But RISE was built on belief acceptance—the understanding that we can't heal what we reject. Instead of fighting our present reality, we meet it with compassion. Instead of demanding instant transformation, we honor timing and biology. Instead of judging our emotions, we learn to listen to them as messengers.

Belief acceptance doesn't mean complacency; it means alignment. It's the act of saying, "This is where I am, and from here, I can grow." In psychological terms, it shifts the nervous system out of threat mode and into a state of safety—the only environment where genuine healing can occur. The group felt the difference immediately. People who had spent years in cycles of guilt began to soften. They discovered that acceptance, not punishment, creates sustainable change.

Embodiment followed naturally. We didn't just talk about wellness; we practiced it. We ate mindfully, breathed intentionally, moved gently, and rested deliberately. We didn't worship discipline; we practiced discernment. RISE became a living, breathing rhythm. The difference was visible—people's faces changed, voices relaxed, laughter returned. They weren't performing wellness; they were inhabiting it.

Early Online Presence and The Rise of RISE

Around this same time, my writing gained momentum. The Healthy in Heart website became the digital home for RISE. What started as health articles evolved into reflections on wholeness, psychology, faith, and food freedom. Each piece ended with practical steps and compassionate questions, inviting readers to participate rather than consume.

Social media amplified the reach. The more stories people shared, the clearer the pattern became: RISE resonated because it gave language to what so many already sensed—that wellness without connection is empty, and spirituality without embodiment is abstract. The philosophy crossed denominational and cultural lines because it wasn't about doctrine; it was about design—the Creator's design for whole-being living.

Handwritten letters and emails began arriving from readers across states and even countries, each echoing the same sentiment: "I thought I was broken, but this helped me see I'm just out of rhythm."

Those words became the heartbeat of the movement. People weren't looking for perfection; they were craving permission—to rest, to eat in peace, to be human again.

Gathering with Intention

As the group found its rhythm, our gatherings became more intentional. Each week we met to explore a new topic connected to whole-being wellness: health, community, spirituality, relationships, food, or emotional balance. Before each meeting, I prepare a set of reflective questions to guide our conversation. One by one, we take turns responding, sharing personal insights and experiences. I usually go first, not as a teacher, but as a participant—modeling openness and honesty so others feel safe to do the same.

What unfolded was more than a discussion; it was a connection. Every question invited awareness, every story revealed common ground. Over time, we began to see patterns—how our choices, thoughts, and beliefs interwove through every aspect of our well-being. Some nights the conversation was light and laughter-filled; other times it was deep, raw, and healing.

The RISE Circle became a space where no one had to have it all together. It wasn't therapy, yet it was deeply therapeutic. It wasn't a church, yet it was sacred. Each gathering reminded us that balance is not a finish line but a practice—a rhythm we can return to, together.

The Phoenix Spreads Her Wings

As the community grew, I often returned to that phoenix image. I began to see RISE not just as my rebirth but as a collective one. Each person who joined the movement was their own phoenix—emerging from the ashes of burnout, shame, or disconnection. Our stories were different, but the fire was the same: a holy hunger for wholeness.

One evening during a group call, someone said through tears, "It feels like we're rising from the ashes together." Her words pierced me. That was precisely it. RISE was no longer mine; it belonged to everyone willing to rise. We weren't escaping our pasts; we were using them as fuel. Every hardship became tinder for transformation. Every scar shimmered like gold in the light of community.

The Embodied Difference

Traditional wellness programs often focus on achievement—lose the weight, hit the goal, manifest the dream. RISE focuses on embodiment. Embodiment asks: *Can you live this truth in your body today?* It doesn't measure progress by metrics but by mindfulness.

Are you present when you eat, breathe, move, pray, rest?

Are you listening to what your body, mind, and spirit are saying?

Embodiment transforms knowledge into wisdom and theory into experience.

Within our community, this looked like small but powerful acts:

- o People pausing mid-sentence to breathe and think deeply before responding.
- o Participants journaling before meals instead of counting calories.
- o Members replacing "I have to" with "I choose to."
- o Whole families shifting from screen-filled evenings to shared walks.

These weren't grand gestures; they were sacred recalibrations. Embodiment that anchored transformation into reality. The philosophy was no longer abstract—it was alive.

The Moment I Knew

I'll never forget the night I realized RISE had become a movement. It was late, the kind of quiet that hums after a meaningful conversation. Our Zoom call had ended, but I sat staring at a black screen that was in my mind's eye still filled with smiling faces frozen mid-goodbye. In that silence, tears came. For years, I had fought alone—for health, for truth, for freedom from shame. Now I was surrounded by others walking the same path. The phoenix had spread her wings.

The fire that once threatened to consume me had become light for others. And I knew: this wasn't the end of healing—it was the beginning of balance. The framework that once saved my life was now shaping lives far beyond mine. It was humbling and holy all at once.

The Philosophy in Practice

From that point, everything evolved naturally. The four anchors became the foundation for books, journals, and teachings. Each resource wove together science, psychology, and spirituality into one cohesive rhythm. We stopped chasing "transformation" and started practicing renewal.

I started to view healing like gardening:

- o Rooted—prepare the soil through truth and grounding.
- o Intentional—plant seeds through deliberate habits.

- o Strong—nurture growth through patience and resilience.
- o Energized—harvest joy and share it freely.

The cycle repeats endlessly, because growth is never finished. The phoenix rises, rests, and rises again.

Carrying the Flame Forward

Looking back, I see how every mentor and moment led here—Karen's guidance, my mother's quiet wisdom, my Cherokee roots, Ross K. Nichols' insistence on honest inquiry, the physicians' science, the community's faith. Each contributed a spark. RISE is the ignition of those sparks into flames—science, spirit, story, and surrender converging into one luminous whole.

And like the phoenix, the work continues. Every circle, every book, every conversation reignites the embers of hope in someone else. The rising never ends; it evolves.

Reflection Prompt

What healing within me might someday serve someone else?

Think of a pain you've carried, a challenge you've overcome, or a lesson you're still learning. How might that experience—your own fire—become a light for others? Write freely, without censoring, and trust that your ashes hold the seeds of someone else's restoration.

PART II

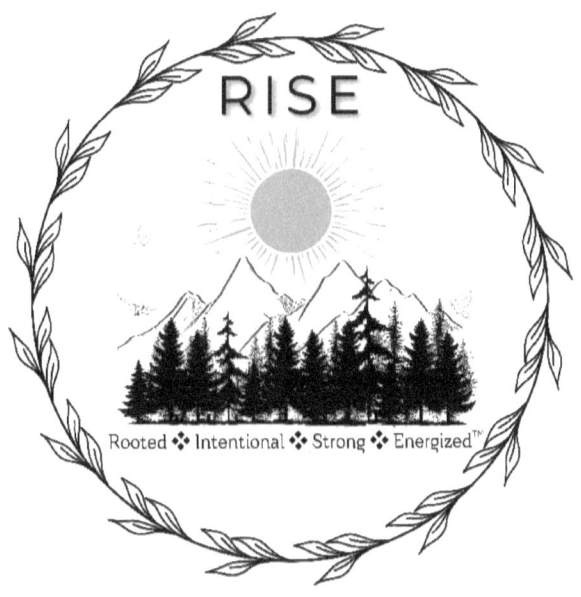

The Longing for Balance

Every human heart carries a quiet ache for equilibrium. We may call it peace, wholeness, or stability, but beneath every label lies the same yearning—to live in harmony with ourselves and the world around us. Modern life rarely honors that desire. Our schedules expand while our spirits shrink; our minds race while our bodies beg for rest. We trade presence for productivity, connection for convenience, rhythm for speed. Eventually, the imbalance manifests everywhere—exhaustion in the body, anxiety in the mind, and apathy in the spirit.

This section explores what that ache really means. Balance is not a finish line; it is a living rhythm, the dance between inhale and exhale, effort and ease, speaking and listening. When one side dominates, we lose the music. The longing for balance is the body's way of reminding us that we were designed for flow, not frenzy.

Here, we examine how imbalance originated, its manifestations in our culture, and how to restore a gentler pace. We will redefine balance as harmony in motion—a dynamic relationship between grounding and growth, purpose and pause. You will recognize the symptoms of disconnection in your own story and learn to interpret them not as failure but as feedback.

The invitation is simple: listen. Listen to the fatigue that says "slow down," to the anxiety that whispers "breathe," to the hunger that asks for nourishment deeper than food. The longing for balance is sacred; it is the voice of creation within you calling you home.

Chapter 7 — The Ache for Balance

Burnout doesn't announce itself politely; it creeps in wearing the disguise of productivity. For years, I thought I was thriving. I had purpose, deadlines, and a to-do list that proved I mattered. But behind the checkmarks, my body was pleading for mercy. Every morning began with coffee and cortisol, every night ended with screens glowing where stars should have been. I told myself exhaustion was a badge of honor—proof of dedication.

It was actually evidence of disconnection.

When Doing Became a Distraction

I can trace my slide into burnout to a season when I confused movement with meaning. If I could stay busy enough, I wouldn't have to feel the emotional pain still pulsing under my skin. I filled every silence with work—writing, studying, organizing, producing. From the outside, I looked driven; inside, I was hollow. Busyness became anesthesia. It dulled the pain, but also anesthetized the joy.

My body finally staged a revolt. Sleep vanished first. Then came migraines, heart palpitations, and the familiar eczema flaring like warning lights on the dashboard of my soul, and even breathing felt like an effort. I remember standing in my kitchen, my hands trembling, as I realized I had built a life that required me to abandon myself daily to keep up with it. That was the moment balance stopped being optional; it became a matter of survival.

Redefining Balance

For most of my life, I thought balance meant evenness—a perfect distribution of time and energy across every category: family, faith, work, health, service. By that definition, balance was impossible. No wonder I felt like a failure. The thought came to me: "Balance is harmony in motion, not perfection." Harmony allows for movement, for the ebb and flow of seasons. Just as music needs both sound and silence, life requires both effort and ease.

True balance isn't symmetry; it's sensitivity. It listens and adjusts. Some days, harmony means tackling projects with focus; other days, it means resting without guilt. The goal isn't to freeze the scales in place but to stay aware enough to notice when they tip.

The Science of Imbalance

Psychology calls burnout a state of emotional, mental, and physical exhaustion caused by prolonged stress and lack of recovery. Neuroscience describes it as the brain stuck in high alert—amygdala over-activated, cortisol flooding, prefrontal cortex offline. In simpler terms, the alarm never turns off. The nervous system forgets how to exhale.

I learned this firsthand. My body had lost its natural rhythm. The circadian cues that once guided sleep, digestion, and mood were drowned out by artificial light and constant stimulation. My phone was the first thing I touched each morning and the last glow I saw before bed. Digital noise became the soundtrack of my life, and silence—real, restorative silence—felt almost frightening.

Physically, the imbalance looked like fatigue that no nap could fix. Emotionally, it looked like irritability and brain fog. Spiritually, it looked like disconnection from wonder.

I wasn't broken; I was misaligned.

The Cost of Constant Connectivity

We live in an age that glorifies the grind. Our devices promise connection but deliver fragmentation. Notifications hijack attention. Comparison corrodes contentment. Even rest becomes performative—spa days posted for likes instead of actual recovery. We've mistaken stimulation for satisfaction.

At my lowest point, I realized I had become addicted to noise. Quiet made me twitchy because it mirrored the emptiness I didn't want to face. The moment I tried to slow down, guilt arrived: You should be doing something. Balance demanded detox—from speed, from striving, from the illusion that my worth depended on output.

The Renewal Begins

The first step back toward balance was brutally simple: stop. I cleared my schedule for one weekend and turned everything off— phone, computer, television. At first, the silence roared. Then something miraculous happened: I heard myself think. Underneath the static, a softer rhythm pulsed—the steady beat of life I had been drowning out. I took long walks, cooked slowly, journaled by candlelight. My mind fought it, but my body sighed with relief.

That weekend taught me what science confirms: the parasympathetic nervous system—our "rest and digest" mode—can't activate amid constant stimulation. Stillness isn't laziness; it's a biological necessity. Balance begins in the body long before it registers in the mind.

Harmony in Motion

Over the next months, I began practicing "micro-balances." If I worked for ninety minutes, I rested for ten. If I spoke for hours, I scheduled silence. If I gave emotional energy to others, I replenished with solitude or nature. These tiny recalibrations prevented collapse. They reminded me that self-care isn't selfish; it's a form of stewardship.

I also redefined productivity. Instead of measuring success by what I produced, I measured it by how present I felt. Presence became the new profit. A balanced day wasn't the one where I checked every box; it was the one where I moved through tasks without losing myself.

Signs of Being Out of Rhythm

Balance rarely disappears overnight; it leaks. It seeps out through skipped meals, chronic tension, irritability, or the inability to feel joy. For me, the red flags were subtle: reaching for my phone the instant discomfort surfaced, eating without hunger, saying "yes" while my gut screamed "no." These micro-betrayals of intuition accumulated until my body screamed for recalibration.

Learning to notice those signals became a form of prayer. Awareness itself was healing. Each symptom was a messenger: fatigue asked for rest, anxiety asked for breath, over-thinking asked for stillness.

Ignoring them was like muting divine guidance.

Cultural Detours

Western culture rarely rewards balance. We admire the hustler, the multitasker, the one who "does it all." But doing it all is often doing too much of nothing that matters. Advertising convinces us that balance can be bought through planners, supplements, and retreats. Yet balance isn't a product; it's a practice. It costs attention, not money.

I began to question cultural definitions of success. Was climbing faster worth losing my peace? Was constant visibility worth constant anxiety? Every "no" I spoke to false urgency became a "yes" to sanity.

The Role of Faith and Surrender

In the stillness, I also rediscovered faith. I realized my burnout stemmed partly from spiritual control—believing everything depended on me. Letting go became worship. Trusting that the world would keep spinning without my constant management freed me to rest. Sabbath, a commandment for a day of ceasing, revealed itself as a rhythm written into creation. Work six days; rest one. Even God paused to breathe as an example for us.

That divine pause taught me a new theology of balance: doing and being are both holy when held in harmony. I didn't need to abandon ambition; I needed to anchor it.

Balance in the Everyday

Balance doesn't require drastic life changes; it thrives in micro-moments. It's choosing water over caffeine, sunlight over fluorescent light, laughter over scrolling. It's remembering to unclench your jaw, to exhale fully, to look at the sky. These small acts restore the nervous system and remind the soul that safety still exists.

I created daily rituals as anchors:

- o Morning light for ten minutes before checking messages.
- o A gratitude note before bed instead of doom-scrolling.
- o Music while cooking to engage the senses.
- o One slow meal eaten without screens.

Each practice rewired my relationship with time. The hours didn't expand, but my awareness within them did.

What Disconnection Has Cost Us

Disconnection costs more than health; it costs humanity. When we lose rhythm, we lose empathy. Overstimulation dulls compassion because we can't feel deeply while moving constantly. Communities fracture, relationships are shallow, and creativity dries. Even spirituality suffers when silence disappears. We start mistaking adrenaline for anointing and applause for purpose.

The ache for balance is therefore not self-centered; it's collective. When one person restores rhythm, it ripples outward. Calm is contagious. Families, workplaces, and communities heal through individuals who model steadiness.

Practical Recalibrations

During this period, I developed a few grounding practices that became staples of the RISE philosophy:

1. The 3-Minute Pause. Three times a day, stop everything, close eyes, inhale for four counts, exhale for six. Let the body reset its rhythm.
2. Digital Sabbath. One evening each week entirely screen-free. Light candles, read, stretch, or talk face-to-face.
3. Rhythmic Movement. Gentle walking, dancing, or stretching synced with breathing—movement that restores rather than drains.
4. Boundary Blessing. Before agreeing to new commitments, ask, "Will this support or steal my balance?"

These micro-disciplines create macro-peace. They aren't about control; they're about cooperation with the body's innate wisdom.

What Renewal Feels Like

Slowly, fatigue lifted. My sleep deepened, digestion improved, and creativity returned. I began to wake with curiosity instead of dread. The simplest moments—sunlight on a mug, laughter shared, a full breath—became holy again. Balance didn't eliminate challenge; it gave me the capacity to meet it. Harmony doesn't erase discord; it teaches how to resolve it.

From Ache to Alignment

Eventually, the longing for balance stopped hurting. It became guidance rather than grief. Whenever tension returned, I treated it as a compass pointing me back to what mattered. The ache itself was mercy—a built-in reminder that wholeness is our default, not our exception.

This realization prepared me for the work ahead. I understood that before we can teach balance, we must live it. Before we can heal others, we must inhabit our own rhythm. The world doesn't need more noise about wellness; it requires living demonstrations of peace.

A Continuing Invitation

Balance will always be dynamic. There will be seasons of intensity and seasons of rest, times to speak and times to listen. But now I know that the rhythm beneath it all is trustworthy. When I forget, the body reminds me; when I drift, creation calls me home. Harmony is not a luxury—it's the language of life itself.

Reflection Prompt

Where do I feel most out of rhythm?

Take a quiet moment. Scan your day like a symphony—where is the tempo rushed, where is there no rest? Write about one small way you can reintroduce pause, silence, or softness. Remember: the ache for balance is not a flaw; it's your built-in invitation to return to harmony.

Chapter 8 — The Moment of Awakening

There are moments in life when everything you've endured suddenly arranges itself into order. Not because the pain disappears, but because you finally understand why it was allowed to exist. For me, that moment came quietly—no trumpet blast, no lightning bolt. Just a steady awareness, rising like dawn: this is what all of it was for.

The healing, the heartbreaks, the endless search for meaning—they were all preparation for what I now know as RISE. It wasn't an idea I invented; it was a revelation I received. One morning, while journaling in my recliner, the four words surfaced again—Rooted, Intentional, Strong, Energized—and this time they didn't feel like reminders. They felt like instructions. A framework had been growing in my spirit for years; I was only now awake enough to recognize its shape.

The Slow Birth of Clarity

Awakening rarely arrives in an instant; it unfolds through layers. Looking back, I can see how each chapter of my life contributed a piece of the pattern. Every imbalance I struggled through—physical exhaustion, one-sided toxic relationships, emotional suppression, spiritual confusion—revealed the anatomy of wholeness by its absence. I had lived the contrast curriculum: learning what health means by losing it, what peace feels like by fighting chaos, and what belonging means by walking through rejection.

For years, I chased answers in books, diets, seminars, and church pews. I was looking outward for what could only be discovered inward. When my body finally forced me to slow down, I began to listen. Beneath the noise of doing, I heard a rhythm pulsing—the same pulse that moves tides, seasons, and breath. It whispered the same truth in a hundred ways: you were made for balance, not burnout.

That was the first tremor of awakening. Not an achievement, but an allowing.

The Sacred Intersection of Pain and Purpose

I often say that revelation is what happens when pain finally meets purpose. My illnesses had taken everything I trusted—my health, my identity, my confidence—and stripped them bare. But the stripping was sacred. It exposed what was real. In the silence that followed burnout, I began to sense that I was being rebuilt from the inside out.

Awakening is not about gaining something new; it's about remembering what was always true. I remembered that my worth was never measured by productivity. I remembered that my body is not my enemy but my ally. I remembered that GOD designed every cell for rhythm and renewal. And I remembered that healing isn't linear—it spirals, looping through the same lessons until they become second nature.

One afternoon, sitting in my garden with my notebook in hand, I wrote the words: Rooted, Intentional, Strong, Energized. I didn't analyze them; I simply let them breathe on the page. When I read them back, something inside me stood taller. The four words felt alive, as if they carried the DNA of everything I'd been learning. That was the moment RISE moved from concept to calling.

Rooted: Remembering Where I Stand

The first word, Rooted, came from the soil of my healing. For years, I had lived uprooted—floating from plan to plan, belief to belief, trying to earn stability through effort. My burnout showed me the cost of living detached from the ground. Rootedness meant returning to what is steady and true: my Creator, my values, my body, and the earth beneath my feet.

Rooted also meant accepting my story—the whole of it. My childhood in Pentecostal holiness, the abuse, the trauma, and also the resilience. For so long, I had tried to escape those parts, thinking healing meant erasing history. But wholeness required integration. Roots don't discriminate between light and dark soil; they draw nourishment from both.

Being rooted taught me to stop striving for worthiness and start growing from grace. It grounded me in truth: that I am not what happened to me, nor what I've achieved, but who I am becoming in relationship with GOD and with life itself.

Intentional: Living by Design, Not Default

The second word, Intentional, emerged from the chaos of distraction. I realized how much of my life had been a reaction rather than a creation. I ate because I was stressed. I worked because I was afraid to stop. I spoke because silence made me nervous. Intention meant reclaiming choice.

Every decision became a sacred act. What will I nourish myself with today—food, words, thoughts, company? Does this action align with the woman I am becoming? I began to treat each yes and no as a brushstroke on the canvas of my life. Even the smallest choices carried spiritual weight.

Intentionality required slowing down enough to listen. The moment between impulse and action became holy ground. That pause—where awareness meets agency—was where transformation truly happened. It was the difference between living life and being lived by it.

Strong: The Courage to Stand and Soften

The third word, Strong, reshaped everything I thought I knew about resilience. For most of my life, "strong" meant hard. HOLD IT TOGETHER. Don't cry. Push through. But my body taught me another definition. True strength includes softness. It bends but doesn't break. It knows when to rest as much as when to rise.

I learned that vulnerability is a form of strength because it allows connection. Setting boundaries is a strength because it protects peace. Asking for help is a strength because it honors interdependence. My nervous system had to learn safety before my spirit could embody power. Strength is not the absence of weakness; it's the presence of grace under pressure.

Through the lens of psychology, strength mirrors self-efficacy—the belief that you can influence your own outcomes. Each time I followed through on a small promise to myself, that belief grew. Confidence didn't arrive as a gift; it was built through daily consistency, one courageous choice at a time.

Energized: The Overflow of Alignment

The final word, Energized, felt like a celebration. For years, fatigue had been my default state—mental fog, emotional heaviness, physical exhaustion. But as I became rooted, intentional, and strong, energy began to return —not as caffeine highs, but as calm vitality. This was not the frantic energy of striving; it was the quiet electricity of alignment.

I realized energy is less about what you consume and more about what consumes you. Worry drains faster than work. Resentment exhausts faster than exertion. When I began releasing what wasn't mine to carry, life flowed through me again. Creativity reignited. Joy resurfaced. The same body that once felt like a cage became a conduit.

This was the final revelation: Energized isn't a mood—it's the fruit of living in rhythm with truth. When we are aligned, energy renews itself.

The Awakening Expands

Once I recognized the four anchors, everything I'd been teaching through Healthy in Heart snapped into focus. I saw how the framework wasn't a theory I built; it was a map of how creation itself operates. Trees root deep into the ground and grow tall with intention toward the light; they strengthen through wind and weather, and energize the ecosystem around them. The same rhythm runs through the human body through seasons and through spiritual growth.

RISE was never meant to be a new system; it was a mirror for an old truth—the ancient pattern of renewal embedded in all living things. The awakening was realizing that my personal story mirrored the universal story: death and rebirth, fall and rising, imbalance and restoration.

RISE as Philosophy and Practice

In the months that followed, I began articulating what had been intuitive. RISE became both a philosophy and a lived experience.

Philosophically, it answered the "why" of wellness—why we ache for balance, why healing resists haste, and why wholeness must include belief acceptance.

Practically, it offered the "how"—daily rhythms that ground, clarify, strengthen, and revive.

The philosophy rests on three simple truths:

1. We are designed for **rhythm**. Every cell, hormone, and emotion follows cycles of rise and rest.
2. Healing requires **honesty**. We can't transform what we refuse to acknowledge.
3. **Embodiment** completes knowledge. Knowing truth intellectually is not enough; it must be lived through the body to become wisdom.

Every teaching, every journal prompt, every group conversation grew from these roots.

A Quiet Moment of Recognition

There wasn't a single dramatic moment when everything suddenly clicked. It was quieter than that. We were in the middle of a conversation about burnout, boundaries, and why people so often feel like they are cycling backward instead of forward. I sketched a simple circle on paper and began naming the four movements I kept hearing in everyone's stories: Rooted, Intentional, Strong, Energized.

As we talked, something subtle shifted. Not wide eyes or gasps, but recognition. People began pointing to places in their own lives. "That's where I am right now." "That explains why this keeps coming back." The language gave shape to experiences they already knew but had never quite been able to name. The circle didn't announce answers; it offered orientation.

Later, sitting with that realization, I felt a deep stillness. What I had lived privately was no longer just my way of making sense of things. It had become a shared language—one that helped people see patterns without shame and movement without pressure. RISE wasn't a declaration or a breakthrough moment. It was a mirror. And that felt far more powerful than any dramatic confirmation ever could.

What Truth Imbalance Revealed

Every revelation is born from a question. Mine began with one I didn't want to ask:

Why do I keep breaking down?

The answer was uncomfortable but liberating—because I kept betraying my own design. I had treated myself like a machine, not a living system. My imbalance revealed that I had believed lies about worth, rest, and control. It showed me that peace was never missing; it was buried beneath the noise.

Imbalance is revelation in disguise. It exposes where we've drifted from alignment. The body's fatigue, the heart's restlessness, the mind's overthinking—all are messages calling us back to truth. My burnout didn't make me less spiritual; it made me honest. It stripped me of borrowed beliefs and returned me to what is real: that we are dust and divine breath intertwined, needing both stillness and motion to thrive.

Awakening as Invitation

Awakening isn't a single event; it's an ongoing relationship with awareness. The moment you think you've arrived, life lovingly hands you another lesson. But each awakening expands capacity—capacity to love, to serve, to rest, and to rise again.

For me, that expansion looked like courage to share my story publicly, to teach without perfection, to embody balance in front of others. The fear of being "not ready" faded because readiness itself was an illusion. The only qualification for leading others into wholeness is the willingness to keep returning to it yourself.

Awakening also birthed compassion. I could finally look at others' imbalances without judgment because I recognized my own reflection in them. We're all learning to find rhythm in a world addicted to noise. That shared struggle unites us more deeply than shared success ever could.

The Psychology of Awakening

From a psychological lens, awakening parallels what researchers call self-transcendence—the stage where personal growth moves beyond self-improvement into meaning-making. It's when pain reorganizes itself into purpose, when individual healing becomes service. This shift rewires the brain toward hope and empathy. It strengthens neural pathways associated with gratitude and decreases those linked to fear.

In simple terms, awakening changes how we process reality. We stop seeing life as happening to us and start seeing it as happening for us. Each challenge becomes a curriculum, each imbalance a teacher. This mindset doesn't deny difficulty; it integrates it.

That's why the RISE framework emphasizes awareness over avoidance. You can't transcend what you won't touch. Healing demands intimacy with our own humanity—the courage to stay present with both shadow and light until they reconcile.

Living Awake

The practical outworking of awakening is attentiveness. It's catching yourself mid-habit and choosing differently. It's noticing when you rush, when you numb, when you disconnect—*and responding with curiosity instead of condemnation.* Living awake means walking through each day as both observer and participant.

I began practicing small awareness cues:

- o Asking "What am I feeling right now?" before reaching for food or my phone.
- o Taking one conscious breath before opening an email.
- o Whispering "Thank You" each morning before standing up.

These micro-awakenings rewired the larger ones. Awareness became muscle memory.

Over time, life felt less like a battle and more like a conversation. The Creator was no longer distant; He was present in the pause, the breath, the soil, the sunrise. Awakening wasn't mystical—it was intimate.

The Awakening in Community

When others began to experience their own RISE moments, I saw how collective awakening multiplies healing. One person's peace stabilizes the group; one person's courage gives permission to others. Through each RISE circle meeting: We rise together.

Community awakening is powerful because it replaces comparison with collaboration. No one's further ahead; we're all at different points on the same spiral. The woman learning to rest is just as vital as the man learning to speak up. Each contributes a note to the song of balance.

Watching others awaken deepened my own. It reminded me that truth is communal—it lives best when shared.

The Phoenix Rises Again

If I could paint this chapter, it would be a phoenix mid-flight— feathers glowing, ash still clinging to wings, eyes fixed on new horizons. That's what awakening felt like: not perfection, but propulsion. The ashes of imbalance still dusted my story, but they no longer defined it. They became evidence of what I'd survived, metaphysical scars.

The same fire that once consumed me had become my light source. I learned that awakening is not about escaping the fire; it's about learning to live within the fire without getting burned. The fire of awareness purifies but does not destroy.

Every time I teach RISE now, I carry that image. Each person in the room is their own phoenix, carrying embers of transformation. Our collective rising lights the sky.

Reflection Prompt

What truth did my imbalance reveal to me?

Look back at a season of chaos or exhaustion. Instead of labeling it a failure, ask what it was meant to teach. What belief or boundary needed adjusting? How did that imbalance expose what you value most? Write without judgment. The same fire that once burned you may be refining you into something radiant.

Chapter 9 — Why We Break Down

Before we ever learn how to rise, we must understand why we fall. Most of us don't break down because we are weak; we break down because we've been carrying too much, for too long, with too little safety to rest. Our minds call it failure, but our nervous systems call it overload. Collapse isn't the absence of strength—it's the body's cry for balance.

When I look back at my own seasons of burnout and illness, I can see that my body wasn't betraying me; it was begging me to listen. The fatigue, anxiety, and compulsive habits were not random. They were adaptive—modifications my system used to try to survive when the world felt unsafe. Healing began the moment I stopped asking, "What's wrong with me?" and started asking, "What happened to me?"

The Psychology of Stuck Cycles

Trauma-informed psychology explains that when our experiences overwhelm our capacity to cope, the nervous system adapts by freezing, fighting, fleeing, or fawning. These protective responses keep us alive in the short term but imprison us in the long term. Many of us live decades later, still reacting to stress as though the danger never ended.

The cycle looks like this:

1. Threat — real or perceived.
2. Response — fight, flight, freeze, or fawn.
3. Relief — temporary sense of safety.
4. Trigger — something reminds the system of the old threat, and restarts the loop.

If the body never learns it is safe, it can't leave survival mode. That's why even after we change our circumstances, we often stay stuck. The body remembers what the mind tries to forget.

In my own story, I spent years in chronic hypervigilance—planning, fixing, controlling. I called it being "responsible," but it was actually fear wearing the clothes of discipline. Overcontrol is the nervous system's way of saying, "I don't trust I'll be safe if I let go." Control feels like power until it becomes a prison.

Overcontrol, Shame, and Survival

Overcontrol is often born from early chaos. When childhood felt unpredictable, when health problems felt like insurmountable mountains, when relationships were out of balance—emotionally, mentally, physically, or spiritually—we learned to manage the environment by controlling ourselves and sometimes also those around us. If we were quiet enough, perfect enough, helpful enough, maybe we'd stay safe.

That coping pattern doesn't disappear with age; it matures into perfectionism, people-pleasing, chronic self-criticism, rigid self-monitoring, emotion suppression, hyper-independence, over-functioning, and yes, sometimes manipulating others.

Manipulating others needs clarity: most trauma-adapted people aren't intentionally manipulative. Manipulation is often a survival strategy—a learned way of managing others' emotions, reactions, or expectations to prevent conflict, avoid abandonment, or maintain a sense of control. Still, the impact is real. I've lived it, seen it, and had it done to me. Overcontrol doesn't just shape who we become; it also shapes how we relate, protect, and sometimes how we harm others.

Shame fuels this cycle. It whispers, "You're not enough unless you fix it all." But shame is not a motivator; it's a silencer. It freezes growth by convincing us that we *are* the problem, rather than recognizing that we *have* a problem.

Some trauma specialists explain that the body often holds the memories our conscious mind can't fully process. When that happens, shame becomes the mind's attempt to explain sensations it doesn't understand. A racing heart, a tightening stomach, a sudden rush of heat—these aren't signs of weakness or failure, though the brain may tell that story. They're protective responses, the body doing its best to keep us safe, even long after the danger is gone.

When Safety Disappears

At the root of every breakdown is the loss of safety. Safety isn't just physical—it's emotional, relational, spiritual. It's the sense that I can be myself and still belong, still be accepted just as I am. When that's missing, the nervous system never entirely rests.

I didn't realize how unsafe my body felt until I tried to slow down. The moment I stopped rushing, panic surfaced. Stillness felt dangerous because my body associated quiet with vulnerability. For years, chaos had been my comfort zone. Healing meant retraining my body to believe peace is safe.

Safety doesn't come from affirmation alone; it's built through consistency. The nervous system learns safety through repetition—steady breathing, predictable routines, trustworthy relationships. That's why small habits like journaling, gentle stretching, or morning light exposure matter. They teach the body a new pattern: "See, we're okay now."

Belief and the Biology of Healing

Our beliefs directly influence physiology. Neuroscience reveals that perception influences biology; our beliefs about our situation can either trigger or calm the stress response. If we believe we're trapped, cortisol surges. Whereas if we think we have a choice, parasympathetic calm increases.

This is where faith and science harmonize. The body responds not just to what's true but to what feels true. That's why healing requires belief alignment…not religious performance, but internal agreement. When my theology said "God loves me," but my nervous system felt unsafe, my body believed the fear, not the verse.

True faith is embodied. It's when the mind, heart, and body agree: I am safe, I am loved, I can rest. That's when healing chemistry begins to flow—oxytocin rises, inflammation lowers, and the immune system stabilizes. The Creator designed the body to respond to truth; our job is to remove the lies that block that signal.

The Nervous System Knows

Your nervous system is not your enemy; it's your interpreter. It translates the world into sensation long before logic comes into play.

- o When your chest tightens, it's not weakness—it's protection.
- o When you overthink, your brain is scanning for safety.
- o When you feel numb, your body is conserving energy.

Learning to decode these signals is the foundation of transformation. The goal isn't to silence the body, but to listen long enough that it stops screaming.

The nervous system knows the truth before the tongue can speak it. Listen with compassion.

How We Lose Connection to the Body

Many of us were taught to distrust bodily wisdom. We spiritualized denial: "Just pray harder," "Don't feel that way," "You're fine." But ignoring sensation is not sanctification.

Disconnection from the body is disconnection from the truth. The nervous system operates on felt experience, not religious slogans.

When we suppress emotion, the energy doesn't vanish; it internalizes. Suppressed anger becomes inflammation. Unacknowledged grief becomes fatigue. Repressed fear becomes control. The body keeps score not to punish us, but to preserve us. It records what consciousness cannot handle in the moment and holds it until we're ready to process.

Reconnection begins with permission to feel. Feelings are data, not directives. You can observe them without obeying them. As we learn to witness sensations with curiosity, the nervous system begins to trust us again.

The Four Stages of Transformation

Through both my personal journey and community work, I began to notice a pattern in how people transition from survival to wholeness. Transformation doesn't happen all at once; it unfolds in four stages—Awareness → Acceptance → Alignment → Embodiment.

1. Awareness: Seeing Without Shame

Awareness is the first crack of light. It's the moment we recognize that something isn't working. Most people stop here because awareness without compassion feels unbearable. But awareness is neutral—it's observation, not accusation. It's the realization that the way we've been surviving no longer serves us.

For me, awareness began when I finally admitted that my health problems weren't random; they were messages. The migraines, anxiety, and cravings were my body sending message after message that I was out of balance. Seeing that clearly was the beginning of choice.

2. Acceptance: Honoring What Is

Acceptance is not resignation; it's recognition. It says, "This is where I am, and I am going to stop fighting reality." Psychologically, acceptance regulates the nervous system because resistance keeps us in a state of fight-or-flight. Spiritually, it mirrors surrender—the peace that comes from admitting we can't heal through control.

This step was the hardest for me. I wanted to jump from awareness to fixing. But healing demanded I sit in the truth without running. Acceptance taught me that discomfort isn't punishment; it's preparation.

3. Alignment: Living from Truth

Once we accept where we are, we can align with what's real. Alignment means bringing belief, behavior, and biology into coherence. It's when your thoughts align with your values, your actions reflect your purpose, and your body feels in harmony with both.

In this stage, you begin setting boundaries, selecting nourishment, and establishing rhythms that reflect your values. You stop forcing and start flowing. Alignment doesn't remove challenge; it clears confusion.

4. Embodiment: Becoming the Lesson

Embodiment is where knowledge turns into wisdom. It's when truth is no longer something you understand but something you are. You no longer have to think about grounding or self-care; your nervous system naturally returns to a state of safety. Embodiment is a transformation that is stabilized.

This is also where service begins—what you've embodied, you can now model. The RISE framework itself was born at this stage of my journey. Once I lived the rhythm of Rooted, Intentional, Strong, and Energized, it began expressing itself through everything I did.

The Dance Between Psychology and Spirit

Modern neuroscience validates what ancient wisdom has always known: renewal begins with rhythm. Every thought pattern has a physiological echo, every prayer a biochemical counterpart. Gratitude rewires the brain for joy; forgiveness lowers blood pressure; meditation repairs neural circuits damaged by stress.

What psychology calls neuroplasticity, Scripture calls renewal of the mind. The body is not secular; it's sacred. Healing is not outside faith—it is faith made flesh.

Understanding this connection freed me from false divisions. I no longer had to choose between therapy and prayer, science and spirit. The Creator authored both. Therefore, balance meant honoring both.

Recognizing Survival Mode in Daily Life

Survival doesn't always look dramatic; sometimes it looks like competence. The one who always organizes, fixes, rescues—that's survival wearing productivity's mask. The one who jokes through pain—that's survival through humor. The one who avoids conflict—that's survival through appeasement.

We survive in the ways that once kept us safe. The problem arises when those strategies outlive their usefulness. What saved you as a child can suffocate you as an adult. Recognizing that...is not betrayal of the past; it's honoring your evolution.

Healing begins when you thank those old strategies for their service and then let them go. You can say: "Thank you for protecting me when I needed you. I don't need you in the same way anymore."

Creating Safety for Transformation

Transformation requires safety because the body cannot grow under threat. This is why healing environments—supportive relationships, calm spaces, gentle language—matter as much as the methods used. Safety is the soil; truth is the seed. Without one, the other cannot root.

When we feel safe, the brain reopens to learning. That's when awareness blossoms into change. This is the psychology behind the RISE Circle: communal safety creates personal transformation. We heal faster together because co-regulation is wired into our biology. Co-regulation is our nervous system syncing through trust.

Each time we sit in honest conversation, share our struggles, or practice mindful breathing as a group, our hearts literally sync. Science calls it cardiac coherence; I call it shalom in motion.

Why We Break Down—and How We Rise

We break down because the pace of life violates the pace of healing. We chase certainty instead of curiosity, performance instead of presence. We ignore the body's wisdom until it speaks through pain. We abandon rest and call it commitment. But the breakdown is not the end of the story—it's the body's way of initiating transformation.

Every symptom is a sacred messenger.

Fatigue says, "You're doing too much."

Anxiety says, "You're carrying what isn't yours."

Depression says, "You've disconnected from meaning."

The invitation is not to silence these voices but to translate them. The nervous system doesn't use words; it uses whispers and waves. When we learn to listen, we learn to rise.

The Integration of the Four Stages

As I began teaching the four stages—Awareness, Acceptance, Alignment, Embodiment—I watched lives change. People who had spent decades cycling through shame finally understood their patterns weren't personal failures; they were protective adaptations. Once safety replaced self-condemnation, healing accelerated.

One woman said, "It's like my body finally exhaled." That's the essence of transformation—the exhale of relief after years of holding your breath. Awareness opens the window; acceptance lets in air; alignment rearranges the room; embodiment lives in it freely.

The Gift of Breakdown

If I could rewrite the story of my own collapse, I wouldn't erase it. The breakdown revealed everything false—false strength, false control, and false self. It stripped me of performance and returned me to presence. In the ashes of exhaustion, I met the truth: I am not a machine to fix but a garden to tend.

The gift of breakdown is that it brings us back to dependence—on God, on grace, on rhythm. When I surrendered striving, balance found me. The body, like the soul, knows how to regenerate when given the right conditions.

Reflection Prompt

What truth did my imbalance reveal to me?

Ask your body what it's been trying to say. What symptom, habit, or emotion might be carrying a message? Which of the four stages—Awareness, Acceptance, Alignment, or Embodiment—are you currently living in? Write honestly, and listen without fear. The nervous system already knows the way home; it only needs your cooperation.

Chapter 10 — The Myth of Modern Balance

We live in a world that worships the busy. The modern gospel of success preaches that the harder we hustle, the more we matter. We measure worth in numbers—steps walked, dollars earned, followers gained, boxes checked. And when our bodies or spirits finally rebel, we call it failure. But what if the real failure is the system that taught us balance could be achieved by performance?

Balance has become a marketing slogan rather than a lived experience. Wellness is sold in neatly packaged trends promising control: track this, buy that, manifest more. Yet the more we chase equilibrium as an achievement, the more elusive it becomes. Balance, by its very nature, can't be forced—it must be felt. The modern world, in its obsession with metrics, has forgotten how to feel.

The Culture of Constant Doing

From childhood, we're praised for productivity: gold stars for perfect attendance, awards for extracurriculars, applause for overextension. Rest rarely receives recognition. The unspoken message is clear: your value is proportional to your visible effort.

As adults, that message mutates into busyness as identity. We wake with alarms, sprint through commutes, multitask meals, and end the day scrolling in exhausted distraction. "How are you?" has become a contest of who's more tired. We wear burnout like a badge of honor and call it ambition.

But beneath the surface, something sacred is breaking. Our souls were never designed for constant acceleration. The nervous system that once responded to a predator in the woods now faces a thousand micro-threats—emails, deadlines, social media comparisons—without pause to recover. The result is a collective dysregulation: anxiety, insomnia, chronic fatigue, and emotional numbness.

We call it normal. It isn't. It's the body's rebellion against a culture that confuses motion with meaning.

Productivity as a Measure of Worth

In modern society, worth has been outsourced to output. We no longer ask, "Who are you?" but "What do you do?" The question itself reveals our disconnection. When being becomes secondary to doing, identity fractures.

I remember the season when I believed this myth most deeply. After launching Healthy in Heart, I poured every ounce of energy into content, schedules, and deadlines. I told myself it was my purpose. In reality, I was terrified of stillness. Productivity was my proof of belonging. If I stayed busy enough, maybe I'd earn the right to rest.

But rest isn't a reward; it's a requirement. The Creator modeled it from the beginning—six days of creation, one day of pause. Sabbath was never about restriction; it was about rhythm. Modern life has severed that rhythm, replacing divine pace with digital pressure. We're always on, yet never truly alive.

This performance-based existence spills into wellness, too. We track calories, steps, mindfulness minutes, even hours of sleep, converting sacred care into a competitive sport. The irony is painful: we're stressing ourselves to the point of exhaustion in the name of self-care.

The Performance of Wellness

The wellness industry, although well-intentioned, often mirrors the same perfectionism that contributed to the imbalance. Smoothies, supplements, and skincare routines become another to-do list, another chance to prove adequacy. The narrative shifts from "I must succeed" to "I must heal," but the underlying desperation remains.

True wellness is not performative—it's participatory. It's not what we post; it's what we practice when no one is watching. It doesn't flaunt perfection; it fosters presence. The RISE philosophy calls this shift the movement from performance to practice.

- o Performance says: "If I do this right, I'll be enough."
- o Practice says: "I am enough. So, I can do this gently."

Performance focuses on optics; practice focuses on embodiment. One drains energy; the other generates it. The difference is subtle but life-changing.

The Psychology of Comparison

Comparison is the invisible thief of balance. It doesn't just rob us of joy; it distorts the truth. Social media amplifies this distortion by offering constant curated glimpses of other lives—bodies, homes, success stories—all filtered through the illusion of perfection. We compare our behind-the-scenes to everyone else's highlight reel, then wonder why peace feels impossible.

Psychologists call this social comparison theory. The human brain, wired for connection, naturally seeks benchmarks to understand belonging. However, in a digital world, without context, comparison can morph from motivation into misery. Each scroll becomes a microdose of inadequacy.

I once spent hours comparing my progress to that of others in the health space—writers, teachers, speakers, and others on the journey. Instead of inspiration, I felt depletion. Then, one day, during a journaling session, I wrote: Comparison kills curiosity. That sentence became a mirror. The moment I measured my growth against someone else's timeline, I stopped learning from my own.

Comparison shifts our gaze outward when balance requires looking inward. Healing happens not when we mimic others but when we honor the unique rhythm of our own becoming.

The Cost of Constant Visibility

Modern culture equates being seen with being significant. The pressure to "show up" online, to brand every experience, to produce constant content, creates a chronic identity crisis. We begin performing our lives instead of living them.

Visibility without vulnerability becomes performance; visibility with vulnerability becomes ministry. The difference lies in motive.

Am I sharing to connect or to control how I'm perceived? The first nourishes; the second depletes.

During the early years, before the RISE philosophy had revealed itself, I felt that tension daily. People looked to me for leadership, wisdom, and consistency. I wanted to be authentic, but I also feared letting anyone see me tired or unsure. Eventually, the mask cracked under its own weight. The day I shared openly about my struggles with fatigue and emotional eating, messages poured in—not of judgment, but relief. My imperfections permitted others to exhale. That's when I realized authenticity is alignment.

From Comparison to Connection

The antidote to comparison is connection—first with ourselves, then with others. Connection requires slowing down long enough to listen. When we reconnect internally, we stop seeking validation externally. Presence replaces performance.

Connection is also contagious. When we model wholeness instead of perfection, we invite others to rest. This is how the RISE Circle became a space of genuine transformation: it was built not on authority but on authenticity. Each person's honesty created safety for someone else's truth.

The Philosophical Root of the Myth

Philosophically, the myth of modern balance was born from dualism—the ancient belief that body and spirit are separate, that work is holy, and rest is indulgent, that doing is masculine and being is feminine. This split still echoes through Western culture, driving us to compartmentalize rather than integrate.

But balance, in its truest sense, is union. It's the reconciliation of opposites: masculine and feminine, action and rest, heaven and earth, science and spirit.

In Hebraic thought, wholeness (shalom) isn't stillness—it's integration: every part of life in right relationship with every other part. Modern culture, in its obsession with extremes, has forgotten the middle way, the way of balance.

When we equate productivity with virtue, we dishonor the divine design of rest. The very systems we built to make life easier— technology, commerce, convenience—now enslave us to pace. We've mistaken tools for masters. Awakening begins when we remember that we were created not for constant output but for meaningful rhythm.

How the Myth Manifests in Daily Life

You can recognize the myth of modern balance in your own day by noticing its mantras:

- o "If I don't do it, it won't get done."
- o "I'll rest when things slow down."
- o "I should be further along by now."
- o "Everyone else is handling it better."

Each phrase reflects a hidden belief: I must earn peace. That belief fuels chronic stress. It's the same mindset that keeps us scrolling for solutions, dieting for worth, and praying for permission to stop.

Breaking that cycle begins with awareness. When you hear those phrases internally, pause and replace them with truth:

- o "Some things can wait."
- o "Rest helps me go farther, not slower."

- "My timeline is sacred."
- "Peace isn't earned; it's remembered."

The nervous system responds instantly to this reframing. The shoulders drop, the breath deepens, the body begins to trust again. Words, when aligned with truth, become medicine.

The Spiritual Cost of Overdoing

Overdoing is not just physical exhaustion; it's spiritual disconnection. In chasing more, we lose the wonder of enough. Our prayers turn transactional: "God, help me accomplish," instead of relational: "God, help me abide."

In the Garden of Eden, work and rest coexisted. Adam tended creation within communion. Labor was never meant to replace intimacy. The curse of modernity is that we've made achievement our god. We seek identity in outcomes rather than in presence.

GOD's rhythm still invites us back: six days of creation, one of restoration. Without that cadence, life collapses into chaos. Sabbath realigns us with divine order. Balance isn't new-age luxury; it's ancient obedience.

Returning to Embodied Wholeness

Wholeness isn't found in having it all together; it's found in having all parts together—mind, body, and spirit in conversation. Modern wellness often focuses on image: the appearance of calm, the curated yoga pose, the spotless meal plan. But an image without intimacy is empty. Wholeness asks: "Are you present inside your own life?"

Embodied living reclaims that presence. It means eating slowly enough to taste, breathing deeply enough to feel, and praying honestly enough to be changed. It's not glamorous; it's grounded. The most radical rebellion against the myth of modern balance is to move through your day at the speed of awareness.

That's what the RISE framework teaches. Rooted grounds you, Intentional focuses you, Strong sustains you, and Energized renews you. Each anchor protects against the cultural drift toward disembodied living.

Why Alignment Outlasts Achievement

Achievement is external; alignment is internal. Achievement depends on outcomes; alignment depends on integrity. One feeds ego; the other nourishes soul. When we chase achievement without alignment, success feels hollow. When we pursue alignment, even small steps are meaningful.

Alignment also creates sustainability. You can't burn out on authenticity. When your actions match your essence, your energy replenishes rather than depletes. That's why living in alignment feels peaceful even when life is demanding—it's congruence, not control.

In my own work, alignment meant saying no more often, choosing depth over reach, and trusting timing over timeline. It meant defining success as stewardship, not scale. Ironically, the more I released my achievements, the greater the impact that followed. Peace is magnetic; people are drawn to authenticity because it feels like home.

The Collective Awakening

Something is shifting globally. People are tired of chasing perfection. They're craving presence, simplicity, and genuine connection. The pandemic years intensified this longing, exposing how fragile constant doing really is. When the world paused, many rediscovered what balance feels like: slower mornings, shared meals, silence that healed instead of haunted.

But as life sped back up, we forgot again. The invitation now is to remember deliberately—to carry that stillness into motion. The RISE movement exists for this purpose: to help individuals and communities live awake within a culture of sleepwalking. To prove that balance isn't about doing less or more—it's about doing what aligns.

The myth of modern balance is losing its power, one awakened heart at a time.

A Personal Confession

Even as I write this, I feel the pull of the old myth. The urge to perfect every sentence, to meet deadlines, to measure worth through words. But each paragraph reminds me: this book doesn't need to impress; it needs to embody. Writing becomes worship when it flows from alignment and authenticity, not anxiety.

Every one of us will revisit the myth again and again. It doesn't vanish; it transforms from master to messenger. When I catch myself hustling for approval, I pause, place my hand over my heart, and whisper, "Return." That one word realigns everything. Return to presence. Return to peace. Return to who you already are.

Reflection Prompt

Where am I chasing achievement instead of alignment?

Think about one area of life—work, relationships, health, or faith—where performance has replaced presence. What would it look like to release control and return to connection? Write honestly. What fear hides beneath the drive to achieve? How might aligning with truth restore energy where striving has drained it? Remember: alignment doesn't make life easier; it makes it real.

PART III

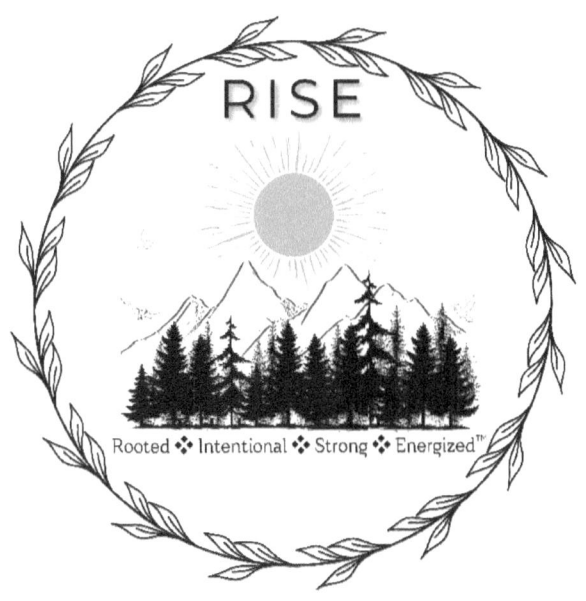

The Framework of Wholeness

Every garden needs fences. Fences are boundaries that protect growth without constraining life. The RISE framework is that fence. It is not a system to master but a rhythm to remember. Each element—Rooted, Intentional, Strong, Energized—mirrors the natural order written into creation itself. When one element weakens, imbalance follows; when all four align, wholeness begins to hum beneath the surface like sap in spring.

Modern wellness often fragments the self, with the body over here, the mind over there, and the spirit somewhere distant. RISE restores integration. It recognizes that healing does not happen in isolation but through the relationship between physiology and faith, thought and emotion, individual and community, creation and Creator.

At its heart, this framework is an invitation to re-inhabit your own life. To slow enough to sense your roots. To act from intention rather than impulse. To cultivate strength that bends instead of breaks. To live energized by alignment, not adrenaline.

Each anchor holds a unique restorative promise:

- o Rooted restores stability—the felt sense of belonging and safety.
- o Intentional restores clarity—living from conscious choice.
- o Strong restores resilience—the courage to remain soft yet steadfast.
- o Energized restores vitality—the overflow of living in truth.

Together they form a circle of renewal, echoing the rhythm of day and night, work and rest, inhale and exhale. To live the RISE rhythm is to remember what the body, soul, and spirit have always known: balance is not a destination; it is the way creation breathes.

We begin where all true growth begins—in the soil.

Chapter 11 — Rooted: Stability in the Soil of Self

A tree cannot flourish if it fears its own ground. Likewise, a person cannot thrive while doubting their right to exist. Rootedness is the quiet confidence that we belong here—that our presence is purposeful, our body is home, and our story has sacred weight.

For years, I lived untethered. My worth rose and fell with external "weather:" praise, progress, productivity, criticism, and backhanded compliments, among others. I mistook motion for meaning, constantly re-potting my soul into new projects, new diets, new ideas. Every uprooting promised transformation, only to leave me more and more depleted. Only when I stopped running did I realize that healing begins not by reaching upward, but by growing downward.

The Ground Beneath the Story

Rootedness begins with remembering where we come from. We are dust and breath—the same elements that form mountains and stars. To be rooted is not merely a metaphor; it is a felt sense of belonging to the created world, of knowing there is ground beneath us even when life feels unstable.

For much of my life, I lived as though that ground were unreliable. I moved quickly, adapted constantly, learned how to read rooms and regulate others before I ever learned how to feel safe inside myself. Psychologically, roots are formed through attachment—the early experiences that teach us whether connection will hold. When attachment is secure, safety becomes instinct. When it is not, survival takes over. I grew up fluent in survival.

As an adult, I kept replaying the same tension in different forms—relationships, work, health, even faith. I thought healing meant going back and fixing what was broken. What I eventually learned was gentler and more hopeful: the task was not to erase the past, but to allow something new to grow out of it.

I often tell people now, "You can plant safety later in life," because I had to learn that truth the hard way. Every time I slowed my breath instead of pushing through, every time I honored a boundary instead of betraying myself, every time I chose presence over performance, something took root. Slowly, almost imperceptibly, my body began to trust the ground again.

Rootedness is not about having had a perfect beginning. It is about cultivating steadiness where there once was strain. It is about letting awareness, compassion, and practice do what time alone could not—send new roots down into the soil of self, until standing no longer feels like bracing, but belonging.

Psychological Safety and the Nervous System

Before purpose and before growth can occur, the nervous system demands safety. When the body perceives threat, the prefrontal cortex—the part of the brain that reasons and plans—goes offline. You cannot think yourself into peace; you must first *feel* safe! Grounding reactivates that safety.

Simple sensory anchors—such as bare feet on grass, slow exhalations, and noticing temperature and texture—signal the body that danger has passed. Over time, these cues rewrite the internal script from "I must brace for impact" to "I can rest and receive."

In RISE language, Rooted is the "restoring" anchor. It teaches stability before strategy. Just as soil nourishes unseen, inner safety sustains everything visible.

Identity: Remembering Who You Are

Rooted identity isn't about titles or roles; it's about essence. When we identify only with what we do, we live in constant fear of loss. But when we remember who we are—a living expression of divine creativity—we find unshakeable ground.

My own reclamation began with three questions:

1. Who told me who I am?
2. Which stories still define me?
3. What truth do I want to root my life in now?

Writing the answers felt like excavation. I unearthed the lies I had learned to answer to:

Too sensitive became compassionate,

Too intense became passionate,

Too idealistic became visionary,

Too different became purposeful,

Too fat became embodied and worthy.

Language matters because roots grow toward what we repeatedly declare.

Spiritually, being rooted means dwelling in a covenant identity: loved, chosen, and created for good works. The Hebrew word for faith, emunah, shares roots with words meaning steadiness and nurture. Faith, then, is not blind belief—it's the stability of trust.

Core Values: The Root System of the Soul

A tree's strength lies not in its trunk but in its unseen network of roots. Likewise, human stability comes from core values—those guiding truths that hold us steady amid shifting circumstances.

When life feels chaotic, returning to values re-centers the nervous system because consistency equals safety. In my own RISE practice, I revisit this simple exercise often:

1. List five values that feel alive for you (e.g., honesty, peace, curiosity, integrity, compassion).
2. Circle the one that feels most neglected right now.
3. Ask: What small action today could water that root?

Values are verbs, not nouns. They must be lived to stay alive. When we practice them daily, identity strengthens organically.

Presence: The Soil of Stability

Presence is the atmosphere that allows roots to breathe. When attention scatters, grounding dries out. I know this not as a theory, but as a pattern I lived for years. My body was rarely where my feet were. I was either scanning ahead, bracing for what might happen next, or replaying what had already gone wrong. Modern life may fracture presence into pixels, but long before screens, my nervous system had learned to stay on high alert.

What changed was not a dramatic breakthrough, but a practice of pausing. I learned to stop long enough to name what was real instead of what was feared. At first, it felt almost too simple to matter:

In this moment, I am safe.

I am breathing.

I am here.

But those words did something my willpower never could. They signaled safety to my body. Slowly, my breath deepened. My shoulders dropped. The constant hum of urgency softened. These moments of presence engaged my parasympathetic nervous system, lowering cortisol and restoring clarity—not because I forced calm, but because my body finally believed it.

Presence also reintroduced me to gratitude, not as positivity, but as grounding. I noticed that anxiety always lived one step ahead of now, while gratitude only existed where my body already was. The brain cannot fully process appreciation and fear at the same time. Each moment of gratitude gently pulled me out of imagined futures and back into embodied reality—the soil where peace actually grows.

Presence did not solve everything at once. But it gave my roots oxygen. And with breath, stability followed.

Grounding Practices

1. **Breathing with the Earth**

    o   Sit or stand with both feet flat. Inhale deeply through the nose, imagining roots extending from your soles into the earth.

    o   Exhale through the mouth, slowly, releasing tension downward.

    o   Repeat for five cycles. With each breath, silently affirm: I am supported.

2. **Journaling Prompt — "What anchors me?"**

    o   Write freely for ten minutes. Begin with the phrase, I feel most steady when...

    o   Notice patterns—places, people, practices that restore calm.

    o   Highlight one anchor you can return to this week.

3. **Sensory Grounding Walk**

    o   Step outside without headphones. Identify five colors, four textures, three sounds, two scents, and one thing that moves. Awareness of sensory detail resets the body's sense of safety.

The Science of Grounding

Research in psychophysiology confirms what ancient traditions intuited: grounding restores equilibrium. Earthing studies show direct contact with natural surfaces regulates cortisol, balances circadian rhythm, and improves sleep quality. But beyond biology, grounding re-teaches belonging.

When you touch the earth, ions exchange, yes—but something deeper happens: you remember that you are part of a living ecosystem, not separate from it. The illusion of isolation, which fuels anxiety and perfectionism, dissolves in that awareness.

Healing from Disconnection

Disconnection is modern exile. We are surrounded by connectivity yet starved for connection. Rootedness heals this exile by reconciling the inner and outer worlds. When we feel safe inside, we stop grasping outside.

During my own healing, I created a daily ritual I called 'Returning to Soil.' Each morning, before checking my screens or schedules, I opened my hands over a small houseplant and whispered gratitude for one thing that had grounded me the day before. It was simple, even childlike, but profoundly re-orienting. My nervous system began to associate mornings with steadiness instead of urgency.

Roots grow through repetition. Stability is not found once; it is practiced daily.

Cultural Lies That Uproot Us

For a long time, I mistook movement for freedom. Culture had taught me that growth meant change, reinvention, and keeping my options open. Staying still felt suspicious. Commitment felt risky. I learned to call uprooting "liberation," even when my body was exhausted from constantly starting over.

We are told that independence is maturity—that needing less means becoming more. I absorbed that message deeply. I prided myself on self-sufficiency, on not asking for help, on adapting quickly wherever I landed. But beneath that flexibility lived a quiet fatigue.

When everything is fluid, nothing feels steady. And when nothing feels steady, the nervous system never fully rests.

Only later did I realize how deeply this contradicted the design woven into every living system. Trees do not thrive by constantly relocating; they flourish by deepening their roots. Underground, they communicate and share resources through mycorrhizal networks. Humans are no different. We regulate through relationships. We stabilize through attachment. Connection is not weakness—it is biology.

Rootedness does not limit growth; it sustains it. What culture framed as confinement turned out to be nourishment. Belonging did not trap me—it steadied me. And steadiness, I learned, is what finally made real growth possible.

Rooted Relationships

The quality of our relationships often reveals the health of our roots. When we are unsteady, we reach for reassurance. When we are grounded, we can offer presence without needing to be agreed with, fixed, or chosen. I have learned this most painfully in the relationship with my sister.

There was a time when I believed closeness meant alignment—that love required mutual understanding, shared language, and staying in step. When distance emerged between us, it shook me more than I expected. Old patterns surfaced: the urge to explain myself better, to prove my intentions, *to restore harmony at any cost.* What I eventually recognized was not a failure of love, but a test of rootedness.

Healthy attachment in adulthood is not fusion; it is interdependence. I am whole, and so are you, and we choose connection where we can. Sometimes that choice includes space. Sometimes it includes grief. Rootedness does not guarantee that relationships will remain intact in the way we hope—it gives us the strength to remain intact when they do not.

Practically, this has meant learning to self-soothe before reacting, to speak honestly without chasing resolution, and to extend grace even when understanding is incomplete. It has meant accepting that I can be grounded in love without being entangled in outcomes.

In community spaces like the RISE Circle, this kind of rootedness creates collective safety. No one has to perform closeness or force agreement. Each person's steadiness enriches the soil we share. And when one relationship feels fragile, the roots we have cultivated elsewhere remind us that we are still held.

Spiritual Grounding

Spiritually, being rooted is about abiding. The psalmist wrote, "He shall be like a tree planted by rivers of water, that brings forth its fruit in its season; whose leaf also shall not wither; and whatever he does shall prosper" (Psalm 1:3, NKJ). Stability doesn't mean stagnation; it means constancy in Source.

Prayer, worship, or simple silence before GOD become acts of rooting. They pull us from surface striving into deep trust. In Hebraic understanding, to "know" God is an experiential process—it occurs through ongoing encounter. Every moment of connection deepens the root of faith.

When the Ground Shakes

Even well-rooted trees face storms. The goal of grounding is not to avoid shaking but to endure it without uprooting. In my own life, crises still arise—health scares, losses, and uncertainty—but the difference now is in their depth. I may sway, but I no longer snap.

When life quakes, return to basics: breath, body, truth. Ask, "What remains steady right now?" Sometimes the only answer is the heartbeat—and that is enough. The same God who steadies the earth steadies you.

Rooted Living in a Disconnected Age

To live rooted in an age of uprooting is revolutionary. It means valuing depth over display, consistency over novelty, and presence over performance. It means slowing when the world accelerates and listening when the world shouts.

Each time you choose grounding over grasping, you resist the myth of instability. You declare that wholeness is not found in constant motion but in conscious dwelling. That declaration, lived daily, becomes your testimony.

Rooted: A Blessing of Belonging

May your roots remember rain even in dry seasons.
May the ground beneath you feel like grace.
May every breath return you to belonging.
And may you know, in marrow and in mind,
that you are planted on purpose.

Reflection Prompt

What anchors me?

List three things—people, practices, or places—that make you feel safe and steady. Describe what each provides: comfort, clarity, courage? Then ask: How can I nurture these roots this week? Stability doesn't come from finding new soil; it comes from tending the soil you're already in.

Chapter 12 — Intentional: Choosing with Clarity

Once you've learned to stand firmly in the soil of who you are, the next step is deciding which direction to grow.

Rootedness anchors; intention orients.

Without it, even healthy roots can sprawl aimlessly beneath the surface, feeding a life that looks busy but feels hollow.

Living intentionally means choosing with clarity—directing energy rather than dispersing it. It is the difference between drifting and steering, between reacting and creating. And like most transformations, it doesn't begin with grand resolutions but with the smallest shift of awareness:

"I will not move unconsciously anymore."

From Reaction to Creation

For many years, I wasn't so much living my life as replaying it. The same emotional scripts surfaced in different settings, relationships, work, and health decisions. The scripts were just dressed in new circumstances. Neuroscience helped me understand why. The brain is designed for efficiency, not wisdom. It relies on patterns formed through repetition and reinforced by emotion. Most of what we do each day happens on autopilot. I certainly did.

When stress or old conditioning took over, my default was reaction. I said yes when my body said no. I pushed through exhaustion and called it discipline. I soothed discomfort with distraction and productivity, mistaking motion for progress. These patterns once protected me. They helped me survive. But over time, they quietly became the very things that kept me stuck.

What began to shift everything was intention—not as a lofty goal, but as a moment-by-moment interruption. I learned to pause and ask, What am I choosing right now? And why? That question alone created space between stimulus and response. A space where choice could breathe.

Psychologically, this is cognitive re-patterning: stepping out of a worn neural groove and forming a new one through conscious awareness. Spiritually, it is repentance in its truest sense—not punishment or shame, but a changing of the mind. Turning toward alignment instead of away from pain.

The RISE philosophy does not treat this process as a form of moral correction. It understands it as liberation. Every intentional choice— no matter how small—becomes a vote for a new pattern. A new pathway. A new way of inhabiting the same life with greater freedom. Over time, reaction loosens its grip, and creation becomes possible again.

Awareness: The First Step Toward Intention

You cannot choose what you do not notice. Awareness is the soil of intentional living. The practice begins with slowing down enough to observe:

- o What am I thinking?
- o What am I feeling?
- o What story am I telling myself right now?

This kind of inquiry shifts brain activity from the limbic system (emotional reaction) to the prefrontal cortex (executive reasoning). The moment you name an emotion or impulse, the amygdala begins to calm. Naming is taming.

Over time, awareness evolves into agency. When you can see your patterns, you can choose differently. That's where intention enters— the bridge between awareness and action.

The Power of Micro-Decisions

I used to believe that transformation required a dramatic overhaul— a moment where everything finally clicked, and I became a different person. What actually changed my life were the smallest decisions, made quietly and repeated long enough to take root.

There were seasons when five minutes of stillness was all I could manage. Days when one nourishing meal felt like a victory. Moments when choosing a calm response instead of sarcasm or self-criticism required real effort. None of these looked impressive on their own. But together, they began to reshape not just my habits, but my sense of what was possible for me.

Neuroscience explains why this works. Each small, conscious choice strengthens a neural pathway. Over time, these micro-decisions accumulate into identity. Behavioral researcher BJ Fogg teaches that tiny habits create significant change because they generate evidence—evidence that the brain uses to update belief. I didn't become consistent because I trusted myself; I learned to trust myself by practicing consistency.

Spiritually, the same principle has always been true. Seeds do not grow because they are dramatic; they grow because they are planted and watered regularly. Intention thrives through faithfulness, not intensity. Again and again, I learned that showing up gently and consistently did more to restore my life than any burst of willpower ever could.

Cognitive Re-Patterning: How the Brain Learns New Rhythms

Our brains are predictive machines. They conserve energy by guessing what will happen next based on past data. This is why change feels threatening; the brain resists new pathways until repetition proves safety. Intention provides that safety.

Consider a familiar pattern: waking and immediately checking your phone. The brain learns to associate dopamine with digital stimulation. Over time, that habit hijacks attention, scattering focus before the day begins.

Now imagine replacing that reflex with the 5-Minute Morning Intention—a RISE micro-practice we'll explore shortly. Each day, you redirect your attention, and the neural network of distraction weakens while the circuit of mindfulness strengthens. After about 30 to 40 days, the new pattern becomes the default. You have literally renewed your mind.

When Proverbs teaches that 'as a person thinks, so they become' (Proverbs 23:7), it's not just philosophy—it mirrors what neuroscience now recognizes about how repeated thoughts shape the brain.

The Myth of Motivation

For years, I waited to feel ready. I assumed motivation would arrive first—that clarity, energy, or confidence would show up and then I would act. What I learned, slowly and repeatedly, is that motivation is emotional weather. It changes without warning. Some days it's bright; most days it's not. Building a life on something so unstable left me stalled more often than moving.

What finally shifted things for me was understanding the difference between motivation and intention. Motivation says, "I'll do it when I feel like it." Intention says, "I'll begin, and my feelings will follow." One is reactive. The other is rooted. Intention became my internal climate—steady enough to support growth even when conditions weren't ideal.

This change was subtle but seismic. Instead of asking, "Do I feel up to this?" I began asking, "What am I choosing today, regardless of how I feel?" That question moved me out of emotional reactivity and into conscious participation. I stopped waiting for permission from my moods and started partnering with myself.

Acting from intention didn't make life effortless, but it made it honest. It returned authorship to my hands. And that, I've come to understand, is sovereignty—not control over outcomes, but stewardship over what is mine to tend, and surrender over what never was. When intention leads, even ordinary days become acts of alignment.

Intentional Living vs. Perfectionism

Intentionality is not another form of control; it's the opposite.

Perfectionism says, If I plan everything, I'll be safe.

Intention says, If I stay present, I'll be guided.

The first constricts; the second flows.

For years, I confused the two. I created rigid schedules and called them "structure." I micromanaged my health and called it "discipline." It wasn't until exhaustion forced surrender that I learned: control is fear's disguise. Intention, however, is faith with direction.

To live intentionally is to plan with open hands—to prepare, not to pressure. It's a conversation with life, not a command.

Mindful Decision-Making: The Three-Second Pause

Every intentional act begins with a pause. Research on emotional regulation reveals that even a brief gap between what we feel and how we respond can significantly alter the outcome. Many psychologists emphasize that this space—however small—is where our choice lives. And in that choice is where growth and freedom begin.

The next time tension rises, take a three-second pause before speaking or acting. Breathe. Ask: "Is this reaction aligned with who I want to be?"

That question transforms confrontation into clarity.

The 5-Minute Morning Intention

This RISE micro-practice rewires the nervous system and primes the brain for conscious living. It's brief enough for busy mornings yet powerful enough to shift the trajectory of your day.

Step 1: Stillness (1 minute)

Sit or stand comfortably. Breathe deeply through your nose for a count of four, hold for four, exhale for four. Repeat. Imagine roots grounding you, just as in the previous chapter.

Step 2: Gratitude (1 minute)

Name aloud or in writing three things you're grateful for—no matter how small. Gratitude changes your brain's default mode from threat detection to opportunity recognition.

Step 3: Intention (2 minutes)

Ask:

- What energy do I want to bring into this day?
- What one quality—peace, courage, compassion—will I embody?

Write it down or say it aloud:

"Today, I choose to move with calm courage."

Step 4: Visualization (1 minute)

Picture yourself living that intention through upcoming moments—meetings, meals, conversations. Visualization activates mirror neurons, preparing the brain to behave as if it were already true.

This five-minute ritual acts as a spiritual and psychological calibration. Instead of reacting to life, you pre-align with it.

Intentional Speech: The Language of Alignment

I didn't arrive at intentional speech because I was naturally positive. I arrived there because my body kept responding to my own words.

During seasons of exhaustion and healing, I noticed that the way I spoke—to others and to myself—either tightened or softened my chest. Phrases I had repeated for years felt factual, but they were quietly training my nervous system to expect scarcity and strain.

When I began experimenting with different language—not denial, but direction—I felt the shift almost immediately. My breath changed. My urgency eased. Over time, I realized that intentional speech wasn't about sounding better; it was about feeling safer. The words I chose served as cues for alignment, signaling to my body and brain where I was headed rather than where I had been.

Words are seeds. They don't just describe reality—they create it. Neuro-linguistic research confirms that language shapes perception; the words you repeatedly use become mental filters.

Notice how often we speak unintentionally:

"I'm so tired."

"I never have enough time."

"This always happens to me."

Each phrase reinforces scarcity, whereas intentional language reframes without denial:

"I'm ready for rest."

"I'll give my time to what matters."

"I'm learning patience through this."

This isn't toxic positivity—it's truth with agency. You're not pretending circumstances are ideal; you're choosing language that aligns with your desired outcome. The nervous system listens.

Intentional Consumption

I learned the power of intentional consumption out of necessity, not discipline. There was a season when my anxiety was loud enough that I could no longer ignore how sensitive my system had become. What I listened to, what I watched, what I ate, and even what conversations I stayed in all left a residue.

I began to notice that some inputs agitated my body while others quietly restored it. That awareness led me to ask a different question—not "Is this allowed?" but "Does this nourish me or numb me?" The shift was gentle but decisive. I didn't overhaul everything at once; I simply started choosing inputs that left me calmer than when I began.

Intention extends beyond what we do to what we absorb. Every input—news, conversation, music, food—shapes internal chemistry. Ask: "Does this nourish or numb me?"

When I began filtering inputs with that question, my anxiety decreased dramatically. I replaced background noise with instrumental music, late-night scrolling with prayer journaling, processed foods with vibrant plants. None of it was rigid; all of it was reverent.

Your body is an ecosystem. What you feed it—mentally, emotionally, spiritually—determines what grows. Be a mindful gardener.

Clarity Through Boundaries

I learned the necessity of boundaries not in theory, but in grief. Setting limits with my sister was one of the hardest decisions I've had to make, not because I stopped caring, but because I finally started caring for myself.

For a long time, I believed love meant endless availability—explaining myself again, absorbing misunderstanding, staying engaged even when my body felt braced and depleted. I overextended myself, took on the responsibility for repairs, and repeatedly forgave and forgot behavior that continued to wound me, particularly in family relationships where shared blood was treated as justification for ongoing harm.

Choosing boundaries felt like failure at first. In truth, it was an act of clarity. I wasn't withdrawing love; I was protecting the conditions required for peace.

Intention requires limits. Without boundaries, energy bleeds into everything. Boundaries aren't barriers; they're irrigation lines. They direct the flow.

If saying yes to everyone else means saying no to yourself, it's not kindness—it's neglect. Boundaries teach the nervous system that you're trustworthy. Each time you honor your "no," your body learns there is safety in self-respect.

Practical boundary setting begins with awareness of capacity. Try this reflection: "What am I giving energy to that doesn't reciprocate peace?" Then decide—gently but firmly—where to prune.

The Spiritual Dimension of Intention

Intention aligns the human will with divine rhythm. It transforms striving into co-creation. When Yeshua prayed, "Not my will, but Yours be done," He wasn't erasing individuality; He was embodying perfect alignment.

To set intention spiritually is to say: "Here I am, use me in harmony with Your design." It turns daily tasks like washing dishes or sending emails into sacred acts of presence.

In Hebraic thought, the word for intention, kavanah, means "directed heart." It implies both focus and devotion. Every intentional choice becomes worship when done with kavanah—a directed heart.

Over time, I learned that spiritual intention doesn't require clarity about outcomes; it requires availability in the present moment. Some days, alignment looks like courage. Other days, it looks like restraint, rest, or quiet faithfulness. When the heart is directed— even imperfectly—life no longer feels fragmented into sacred and secular. There is only responsiveness. Intention becomes the bridge between heaven and habit, turning the ordinary rhythm of a day into a steady conversation with the Divine. Not perfection— participation.

How Intention Rewrites Emotional Memory

I didn't realize how much my past was still choosing for me until my reactions started surprising me. Certain tones, moments of conflict, or even silence could flood my body before my mind caught up. I wasn't deciding—I was remembering. What began to change that pattern wasn't insight alone, but intention practiced in real time. Each time I responded with breath rather than urgency, or paused rather than proving myself, my body logged a different outcome. Nothing bad happened. I stayed safe. Over time, those moments began to accumulate into something new—not just understanding, but emotional memory.

Unhealed emotion drives unconscious choice. Intention breaks that pattern by creating new emotional memories. When you repeatedly act from a place of peace rather than fear, your nervous system learns that safety lies in calm, not chaos.

Over time, what once triggered anxiety becomes a cue for mindfulness. You might even begin to miss your intentional rituals when you skip them—that's how you know re-patterning has taken root. The body starts craving coherence.

From Mindfulness to Meaning

The difference between mindfulness and meaning became clear to me during a season of relational rupture with my sister. I was deeply aware of what I felt—sadness, grief, confusion, the ache of betrayal. Awareness alone kept me tender, but also stuck. I could name my emotions, but I didn't know how to move with them.

What changed was intention. Instead of spiraling in what I felt, I began choosing how I would respond inside it—when to breathe instead of react, when to release instead of rehearse, when to trust that space could still be an expression of love. Awareness showed me what was true; intention showed me how to live with it.

Mindfulness is awareness, and intention adds direction. Awareness notices, "I'm anxious." Intention adds, "I choose to breathe through this moment." Awareness is the open window; intention decides what enters.

Meaning arises when intention aligns with purpose. You begin to sense divine partnership in daily details. Coincidences feel like confirmations. Life no longer happens to you; it happens through you.

The Shadow Side: When Intention Becomes Obsession

I saw the shadow side of intention most clearly in the wake of my sister's betrayal. There were a dozen ways I could have responded that looked intentional but were actually driven by control—replaying conversations to get the wording just right, drafting messages I never sent, rehearsing explanations that might finally make me understood, tightening my grip on outcomes I could not manage. I told myself I was being thoughtful, measured, even righteous. In truth, my nervous system was braced. My body wasn't at peace; it was vigilant. That's when I realized intention had quietly slipped into obsession.

Like any virtue, intention can distort into control. Hyper-focusing on every choice can lead to anxiety or self-judgment. The goal is consciousness, not perfection. A healthy sign you're in balance: peace increases, pressure decreases.

Remember: Intention is not about forcing outcomes but fostering awareness. When uncertainty arises, repeat this affirmation:

"I choose clarity over control."

That phrase instantly brings breath back to the body.

Intentional Community

My understanding of intentional community was forged during seasons when connection felt fragile. After relational fractures—especially within my own family—I became acutely aware of how much the body needs safe, attuned presence to heal. I learned that isolation didn't make me stronger; it made me vigilant. Community, when chosen with intention, did something different. It regulated me. It reminded my nervous system that steadiness could exist beyond a single relationship. The RISE Circle grew out of that realization—not as a replacement for what was lost, but as a place where rooted, intentional connection could be practiced together.

Intention expands in community. When shared aloud, it gains accountability and momentum. In RISE Circles, we will often begin or end a session with a spoken intention. Something shifts in the atmosphere when ten voices declare, "Today I choose presence." The collective nervous system harmonizes.

Science calls this "social entrainment"—our heart rhythms sync with those around us. Spirit calls it an agreement. Either way, intentional unity magnifies healing.

A Day Lived Intentionally

Imagine waking with gentle light filtering through the window. Instead of reaching for your phone, you place a hand on your heart, breathe deeply, and whisper today's intention. You rise slowly, stretch, drink water, and open a journal to write one sentence: "I will move through today with patience and purpose."

As you encounter challenges, you recall that sentence like a compass. At work, when stress surges, you pause for three seconds and respond calmly. During lunch, you taste food instead of scrolling. In the evening, you step outside, notice the sky's gradient, and feel gratitude swell. The day may not have been perfect, but it was present.

That's intentional living: not changing everything, but being awake for what already is.

To live intentionally is to walk as a co-creator with the Divine. Each breath becomes a part in a greater rhythm, and each decision a brushstroke on the canvas of your becoming.

When you live by intention, you no longer chase balance—you embody it.

And from that grounded clarity, strength begins to grow.

A Blessing for Choosing with Clarity

May your choices come from stillness, not striving.
May you learn to recognize the quiet wisdom
that surfaces when you stop forcing the way forward.

May clarity replace chaos,
discernment soften urgency,
and truth steady your steps.

May each small, intentional decision
become an act of trust—
guiding you gently into what is whole and life-giving.

Reflection Prompt

Where in my life am I reacting instead of making a choice?

Write down one pattern—an argument, a habit, a thought loop—that feels automatic. Then, answer: What would conscious creation look like in this context? Define one new intention to replace the old reaction.

Chapter 13 — Strong: Resilience Through Grace

Strength is often misunderstood.

We picture clenched fists, grit, and unbending willpower. Yet the deepest kind of strength rarely looks like striving; rather, it looks like acceptance. It's the quiet courage to remain open when life demands closure, to stay kind when disappointment hardens others, to pause when every instinct screams to push.

Real strength isn't the absence of weakness—it's the presence of grace within weakness.

When I think back to my own seasons of breaking and rebuilding, I see how often I mistook tension for toughness. I equated resilience with resistance, as though bracing harder could keep pain at bay. But every storm that tried to knock me down became a teacher: the trees that survive aren't the stiff ones—they are the ones that bend.

That's what this anchor of RISE is all about: learning to bend without breaking.

Redefining Strength

In a culture that glorifies hustle and stoicism, strength has been distorted into suppression. We admire those who "keep it together," rarely asking what it costs them to hold it so tightly. I felt that cost most acutely during a season when my sister lied about me in court. The accusation itself was so unfounded that even my attorney treated it as absurd, but the impact on my heart was anything but trivial. Being misrepresented by someone bound to you by blood and what was at one time a very close relationship exposes how fragile false definitions of strength really are.

True strength isn't found in never falling apart; it's in learning how to fall apart safely. In that season, I could have hardened myself, retaliated, or proven my innocence with relentless explanation. Instead, strength looked like restraint. It looked like letting tears come without letting bitterness take root. It looked like admitting, I cannot carry this alone, even when I was technically vindicated.

Grace changed the equation. Grace said: Strength isn't earned by endurance alone—it's infused through surrender. The strongest people I know aren't those who never cried; they're those who cried and kept walking anyway. Grace allowed me to let go of the need to be understood by everyone and to trust that truth did not require my overexertion.

In my life, strength has taken the form of getting up after grief, forgiving when resentment would have felt justified, and choosing integrity when self-protection would have been easier. Each time I loosened my grip on control, something met me there—peace that didn't make sense, provision I hadn't orchestrated, renewal I couldn't manufacture. That is grace in motion.

Resilience: The Art of Returning

I didn't learn resilience by staying upright, but by having to return—again and again. There were seasons when disruption felt constant, when my nervous system rarely had time to settle before the next demand arrived. Family strain, grief, disappointment, and the slow work of healing taught me that pushing through only delayed recovery.

What actually rebuilt me was learning when to rest, when to pause, and when to let my body recalibrate instead of forcing forward motion. Resilience, I discovered, wasn't about how much I could endure, but how faithfully I could come back to center after being knocked off balance.

Psychologically, resilience isn't toughness; it's elasticity. It's the nervous system's ability to return to balance after disruption. Emotional resilience develops the same way physical stamina does—through stress and recovery cycles.

Too much stress breaks; too little stagnates. Healing environments offer a balance: enough challenge to foster growth, and enough rest to facilitate integration. This is why safety and intention precede strength in the RISE sequence. Without a grounded identity and clear intentions, effort becomes strain.

Resilience is not about avoiding collapse, but about returning from it quicker and wiser each time. As the body trains through micro-stressors—like lifting weights—it adapts. The spiritual life mirrors this: trials stretch our capacity for faith, but rest rebuilds it.

The key is to honor both phases. Grace is the rest that makes growth sustainable.

Emotional Regulation: Strength of Spirit

One of the most powerful forms of strength is self-regulation—the ability to hold emotional charge without exploding or imploding. When emotions surge, our nervous system floods the body with energy designed for action. Without awareness, that energy spills into reactivity. With awareness, it becomes fuel for growth.

I learned emotional regulation the hard way—by realizing how often I was needed to stay composed in genuinely painful situations. In moments of relational strain, especially within my family, I felt strong emotions rise quickly: anger at being misrepresented, grief over what couldn't be repaired, fear of saying the wrong thing and making things worse. Earlier versions of me either swallowed those feelings to keep the peace or let them spill out in ways that left me drained.

What healing taught me was a third way: to stay present with the emotion without becoming it. Regulation became less about control and more about staying anchored while the wave passed.

Emotional regulation doesn't mean numbing. Emotional regulation means navigation. It's the skill of acknowledging your feelings without being ruled by them. Psychologists refer to this as "affect labeling," which involves naming your emotions to better understand and manage them. Spiritually, it's discernment—learning to recognize which feelings are invitations and which are illusions.

When anger arises, ask: What boundary was crossed?

When sadness lingers, ask: What attachment am I releasing?

When fear speaks, ask: What is asking for reassurance?

Every emotion has a message. Strength is found in listening without losing yourself in the story.

Boundary-Based Courage

I learned boundary-based courage in a season when staying open-hearted required more bravery than retaliation ever would have. When my sister crossed a line that could not be uncrossed—misrepresenting me and trying to tarnish my reputation—I felt the familiar pull to overexplain, absorb, and endure for the sake of family peace. The truth prevailed, but the emotional cost was real. What I faced in that moment was not just betrayal, but a choice: continue abandoning myself in the name of love for her, or let love for myself and courage take a quieter, firmer form.

Healthy boundaries are the backbone of emotional strength. They define where responsibility begins and ends. Without them, empathy turns into exhaustion, and compassion turns into codependence.

I learned this the hard way. For years, I thought love meant self-sacrifice without limit. I absorbed everyone's pain, forgetting that carrying someone's burden isn't the same as taking it away. My healing began when I realized boundaries aren't walls—they're gates. They protect what's sacred while allowing what's safe.

Boundary-based courage says: I will remain open-hearted, but I will not abandon myself in the process.

To set a boundary is to tell the truth about your capacity. It's saying,

> "This is what I can give with love, and
>
> this is where I must rest to keep that love real."

The nervous system interprets boundaries as a sign of safety, not selfishness. Each time you honor one, you reinforce trust in yourself.

The Biology of Grace

I didn't come to understand grace through doctrine alone; I came to it through exhaustion. There were seasons when my inner dialogue was relentless—replaying mistakes, questioning motives, rehearsing conversations I wished had gone differently. Even when I was "right," my body felt unsafe.

What finally interrupted that cycle wasn't more discipline or better reasoning, but compassion directed inward. When I began speaking to myself with the same gentleness I would offer a wounded child, I felt an immediate shift. My breath softened. My shoulders dropped. Grace, I realized, was not just mercy for the soul—it was medicine for the nervous system.

Grace isn't just theological—it's physiological. When you extend compassion to yourself, your body shifts from a state of threat to one of repair. Oxytocin levels rise, cortisol levels decrease, and heart coherence stabilizes. Self-compassion literally heals the stress response that shame creates.

Dr. Kristin Neff's research on self-compassion shows that gentle self-talk activates the same calming systems as a mother soothing a child. This isn't indulgence—it's intelligence. You cannot shame yourself into strength; you can only love yourself into it.

When you fail, whisper grace into your nervous system: "It's okay, I'm learning."

When you're weary, remind yourself: "Rest is resistance, not retreat."

Each gentle thought rewires pathways that once linked effort to fear. That is how grace grows resilience at the cellular level.

"Pause Before Push" — The Practice of Graceful Strength

Modern culture conditions us to push through pain. While persistence has its place, chronic pushing fractures alignment. The body breaks down because the soul has no pause.

The RISE practice of Pause Before Push invites a sacred micro-moment between effort and exhaustion.

Step 1: Notice the urge to push.

You'll feel it as tension in the shoulders, shallow breath, or racing thoughts.

Step 2: Breathe and ask:

Is this push necessary, or is it fear-driven?

Step 3: If it's fear-driven, pause instead of powering through.

Drink water, stretch, pray, or step outside for one minute. Reset your nervous system before resuming.

This habit cultivates embodied discernment. It teaches that you don't lose momentum by pausing; you preserve it. A pause in grace prevents collapse in guilt.

The Strength of Surrender

The paradox of power is that it multiplies when released. In Scripture, surrender never meant defeat—it meant alignment. When Yeshua said, "Into Your hands I commit my spirit," it was the ultimate act of empowered trust. He modeled strength that yields rather than resists.

I learned the strength of surrender in a season when there was nothing left that I could manage. After doing everything I could to act with integrity—telling the truth, setting boundaries, showing up with care—I reached the edge of my own capacity. Outcomes were no longer mine to influence. I could feel the cost of continued vigilance in my body: tight shoulders, shallow breath, a constant readiness to defend. Surrender didn't come as a spiritual epiphany; it came as a necessity. Letting go wasn't weakness—it was relief. It was the moment I stopped trying to hold what was never meant to be carried by me alone.

Surrender is not giving up; it's giving over. It's transferring the weight of outcome from self-effort to divine order. In practical terms, it sounds like:

"I will do what I can with excellence and leave what I cannot do to God."

This posture frees the body from chronic vigilance. Muscles unclench. The nervous system releases its grip. Surrender restores rhythm—the balance between doing and being. Strength becomes sustainable when it flows in this divine alternation.

Resilience Through Community

No one builds resilience in isolation. Just as trees interlock roots underground for mutual stability, humans regulate through connection. When we co-regulate—safely sharing emotional space—our nervous systems synchronize, lowering collective stress.

This is why group support, such as the RISE Circle, accelerates healing. In these spaces, you practice both vulnerability and boundary. You speak your truth and listen to others without taking ownership of their outcomes. Each time you witness another's strength, your own expands.

Grace moves through the community as shared compassion—each person becoming a mirror and medicine to the others.

The Courage to Stay Soft

It takes more strength to stay gentle in a harsh world than to harden with it. Softness is not weakness; it's maturity. The Hebrew word rachamim (mercy) comes from rechem, meaning womb—protection that nurtures and shields. That's the essence of strength through grace: creating safety that gives life, not control that constrains it.

To stay soft is to keep your heart breakable and still believe in beauty. It means choosing compassion over cynicism, empathy over apathy. Such softness is holy defiance—it keeps love alive in a world that profits from division.

Resilience in the Nervous System

Physiologically, resilience requires oscillation between activation and rest. Just as muscles need recovery after weightlifting, emotions need restoration after intense experiences. Practices that regulate this oscillation include:

- o Deep diaphragmatic breathing (lengthening on the exhale activates the vagus nerve).
- o Alternating movement and stillness (walking, stretching, then meditating).

- Journaling emotional charge before responding.
- Prayerful release: audibly exhaling burdens while naming them.

When practiced consistently, these rhythms increase vagal tone—a measure of the body's ability to return to a state of calm. In spiritual language, peace becomes your baseline.

When Strength Feels Like Stillness

There was a moment when every instinct in me wanted to act—explain, correct, defend myself, loudly and angrily. Silence felt risky. Stillness felt like surrendering my voice. But in the aftermath of being misrepresented within my own family, I sensed that an immediate response would only keep the turmoil alive. Choosing not to react was not passive; it was deliberate. It required more strength to wait than to speak. In that stillness, truth had room to stand on its own, and my nervous system finally had space to settle.

Sometimes the bravest thing you can do is nothing. Waiting, listening, letting things unfold—these are forms of active strength. Our culture prizes immediate response, but heaven values patient alignment.

When uncertainty looms, resist the reflex to fix. Sit in the question. Often, clarity arises not from control but from quiet. Like a shaken snow globe, truth settles when you stop shaking it.

Stillness is not stagnation; it's strategic recovery. It's what keeps purpose from collapsing under pressure.

Integrating Past Pain Into Present Power

I didn't set out to integrate pain; I wanted relief from it. But the rupture in my relationship with my sister forced a different reckoning. There was grief I couldn't bypass, betrayal I couldn't reframe away, and a loss of closeness I had to carry without resolution.

What I discovered, slowly, was that pain unexamined kept me braced, but pain brought into the light began to teach. As I allowed myself to grieve honestly, set boundaries clearly, and stop chasing understanding and forgiveness that wasn't being offered, something shifted. The experience didn't harden me—it clarified me. What emerged wasn't bitterness, but discernment. Not distance, but depth.

Every hardship carries hidden wisdom. When processed, pain becomes compost—enriching the soil of your soul. To integrate rather than avoid pain, ask reflective questions:

- o What did this experience reveal about my resilience?
- o How did grace meet me there?
- o What boundaries or values emerged because of it?

Integration turns memory into meaning. It transforms survival into strength that blesses others. We comfort others with the comfort we ourselves have received.

The moment pain gives rise to empathy, it stops being wasted.

Signs You're Growing Stronger

You'll know grace-based strength is forming when:

- o You respond slower and softer.
- o You recover quicker from conflict.
- o You say "no" or "I'm done" without apology.

- o You rest without guilt.
- o You trust timing instead of forcing it.

These shifts are subtle yet sacred. They mark the transition from striving to sovereignty.

The Strength to Begin Again

I came to understand the strength to begin again when I finally stopped pursuing a relationship that existed only on someone else's terms. With my sister, I reached a point of clarity that was both painful and freeing: I could continue reaching, explaining, and forgiving without reciprocity—or I could accept what was being shown to me.

When accountability was refused, when harmful behavior went unnamed and unrepentant, and when repair was expected without responsibility, I realized that continuing to pursue closeness would require abandoning myself. Choosing to stop wasn't bitterness; it was honesty. It wasn't punishment; it was a boundary that allowed healing to move forward instead of circling the same wound.

Every season ends. Every healing cycle closes. The courage to begin again—to re-enter growth after loss—is the ultimate sign of strength. The phoenix rises not because it avoids fire, but because it trusts renewal more than ashes.

That same renewal lives in you. The RISE journey teaches that endurance is not linear progress—it's a circular process of grace. Each time you fall and rise again, the circle widens. You carry more compassion, more wisdom, more peace.

Practice: Pause Before Push

Purpose:

To transform the instinct of overdrive into an embodied pause that restores perspective.

How to Begin:

1. Set an anchor phrase. Choose words that remind you to soften—such as "Grace first."
2. Notice cues of overexertion: jaw tension, shallow breathing, resentment, or mental fog.
3. Pause for one deep breath. Feel your feet on the ground. Exhale slowly.
4. Ask: Am I pushing from peace or from fear?
5. Choose: proceed gently if peaceful; step back if fearful.

Over time, this two-minute pause rewires urgency into trust. It becomes a living boundary between burnout and balance.

Strength through grace is not about conquering life but cooperating with its rhythm. It's the ability to meet a challenge without losing compassion, to hold tension without breaking trust. When you live this way, others feel safer in your presence because your peace has become palpable.

And that is the quiet revolution of RISE: strength that steadies, love that lasts, grace that keeps us standing.

A Blessing for the Strong in Spirit

May your strength be steady, but never hard.

May your boundaries bloom like gardens, not fences.

May you pause before push,

Rest before rupture,

Surrender before shatter.

And may grace be the wind that bends you, not the storm that breaks you.

Reflection Prompt

Where in my life am I mistaking pressure for power?

Identify one area—work, health, relationships—where you tend to "push through." Journal what it might look like to pause before push. How could grace strengthen your resilience there?

Chapter 14 — Energized: The Flow of Alignment

When the roots are grounded, the mind aligned, and the heart resilient, something remarkable begins to happen—energy flows. Not the caffeinated surge that burns out by noon, but the quiet radiance of harmony. It's not adrenaline; it's aliveness. This is the final movement of RISE—the Energized anchor—the phase where wholeness becomes visible.

Energy is rhythm, not overdrive. It moves like breath: inhale receiving, exhale releasing. Alignment keeps this rhythm steady. When energy stagnates, we feel fatigue, irritation, or confusion. When it flows, we feel focused, creative, and deeply present. The purpose of RISE isn't to help you do more—it's to help you live at the natural pace of your own vitality.

Energy as Rhythm, Not Overdrive

In modern culture, "energy" has been hijacked by the productivity myth. We equate high performance with high worth, confusing endurance with vitality. But sustained overdrive doesn't create energy—it consumes it.

I learned the cost of overdrive not through ambition, but through survival. For years, I lived as though staying ahead of exhaustion was the same as being energized. I pushed through emotional strain, family conflict, and chronic stress by tightening my grip and calling it resilience.

My body kept tallying the score. Eventually, the fatigue, fog, and nervous system strain made it clear that what I had labeled "strength" was actually misalignment. I wasn't honoring rhythm; I was overriding it. Healing required more than rest—it required relearning how to live in cadence rather than in constant output.

Biologically, the human body operates in cycles of activity and recovery. The heart beats, then rests; the lungs fill, then release; cells repair during sleep. To remain "on" perpetually is to violate the very design of creation. That violation has consequences: chronic fatigue, adrenal dysregulation, emotional burnout, and cognitive fog.

The rhythm of energy mirrors the rhythm of Sabbath: six days of creative engagement, one day of sacred stillness. When we honor this built-in balance, energy regenerates naturally. When we ignore it, we borrow from tomorrow to survive today.

So, the RISE definition of "energized" is not driven, but in tune. Energy is the byproduct of inner coherence—mind, body, and spirit working together instead of against each other.

Alignment: The Conductor of Flow

Imagine your life as an orchestra. Every instrument—nutrition, movement, thought, emotion, rest—plays a part. When one section dominates or plays out of key, the harmony collapses. Alignment restores the conductor's baton.

I came to understand alignment not as harmony achieved, but as resistance released. For a long time, I spent enormous energy trying to make a relationship work that was no longer meeting me in truth—adjusting myself to accommodate another person who wasn't willing to make any adjustments of her own, hoping for accountability that never came. With my sister, I felt the constant internal dissonance of loving someone while denying what was actually happening. That resistance drained me far more than grief ever did. Alignment arrived the moment I stopped arguing with reality and allowed truth—however painful—to take the lead. My energy didn't disappear; it reorganized.

In neuroscience, alignment corresponds to neural coherence—the brain's networks firing in synchrony. When thought, intention, and behavior align, energy output becomes efficient. The mind stops leaking power through internal conflict.

Spiritually, alignment is agreement with truth. It's living in rhythm with divine order instead of wrestling against it. When you say "yes" to what's real and "no" to what's false, energy stabilizes.

Resistance is one of the greatest drains of life-force—arguing with reality consumes vitality faster than any physical exertion.

So, ask often: Where am I resisting what already is? Acceptance doesn't mean approval—it means conservation of energy for what you can change.

Nutrition: The Physical Flow

My relationship with food changed when I realized how deeply my body was affected by emotional strain. During seasons of stress and relational upheaval, I noticed that what I ate either amplified the noise in my system or helped quiet it. Heavy, processed foods left me foggy and reactive; simple, living foods made me feel more grounded and clear. Nutrition stopped being about control or perfection and became about regulation and respect. Choosing foods closer to their original form felt like cooperating with my body instead of overriding it—an act of alignment rather than discipline.

Food is more than fuel; it's information. Every bite sends biochemical messages to your cells, telling them either to inflame or to heal. When you choose whole, living foods—fruits, vegetables, legumes, grains—you're literally feeding your mitochondria the light they were designed to use. The chlorophyll in plants captures sunlight; when you eat them, you internalize that energy source.

In Edenic design, food was a form of communion with creation. Every color, flavor, and texture carried both pleasure and purpose. Returning to that simplicity reawakens vitality.

Energy drains through over-processed foods, excess sugar, and chemical additives that confuse the body's natural intelligence. As Dr. John McDougall taught: The human body runs best on starch-based, whole foods, not fear-based diets. In my own journey, I learned that the more natural my plate became, the more peaceful my mind felt.

Eating with intention transforms nourishment into gratitude. Before each meal, pause and ask:

"Will this bring me closer to life or further from it?"

That one question aligns body and spirit before digestion even begins.

Movement: Energy in Motion

I learned the necessity of movement during a season when my body felt heavy with unspoken emotion. Stress, grief, and relational strain had a way of settling into my chest and shoulders, leaving me tight and tired even when I was technically resting. What surprised me was how quickly gentle movement shifted that weight. A quiet walk, stretching in the morning light, swaying while listening to worship music—these weren't workouts, but releases. Movement reminded my body that it wasn't trapped. I didn't need to push or perform; I needed to circulate what had been held.

Energy was never meant to stay still. The body is a dynamic ecosystem that thrives in a state of flow. Movement doesn't just strengthen muscles—it circulates lymph, balances hormones, and clears emotional residue stored in the fascia.

In trauma-informed physiology, movement re-establishes agency. Gentle walking, dancing, stretching, or gardening tells the body, I am safe enough to move freely. This is why movement is foundational to emotional regulation—it transforms trapped survival energy into creative expression.

Find your personal rhythm. Some days it might be brisk walking with worship music. Other days, it's slow yoga, grounding barefoot in the grass, or swaying gently to your breath. There is no formula. The question is not "Did I exercise?" but "Did I move in a way that honors the life within me?"

Remember: movement should restore, not punish. Sweat and strain don't sanctify—presence does.

Thought: The Subtle Energy Source

I became aware of the power of thought when I realized how much energy I was losing in my own mind. During seasons of stress and relational rupture, my thoughts ran ahead of me—replaying conversations, anticipating conflict, questioning my own integrity even when I had acted in truth. My body responded immediately. Tight chest. Shallow breath. A heaviness that no amount of rest could fix. What surprised me was how quickly that energy returned when I interrupted the spiral. When I challenged a thought instead of believing it, my shoulders softened. My breath deepened. I wasn't fixing my life—I was restoring my frequency. Thought by thought, I learned that mental alignment wasn't just emotional hygiene; it was energetic stewardship.

Every thought generates electrical activity measurable in the brain. Positive, life-affirming thoughts produce coherent energy; fear-based or self-critical patterns fragment it. This is why alignment at the level of thought is essential to vitality.

Cognitive scientists have shown that gratitude and compassion increase dopamine and serotonin levels, enhancing mood and motivation. Conversely, chronic worry floods the body with cortisol, draining cellular energy.

You can feel the difference instantly. Think of a time you felt inspired—your chest opened, your breath deepened, you wanted to move. Now recall a moment of anxiety—your stomach clenched, shoulders tensed, energy collapsed inward. The mind sets the body's frequency.

Renewal begins with awareness. When you catch yourself spiraling into negative self-talk, pause and replace the thought with something true and empowering. Use the acronym "TRUE":

- o **T**hought – Identify it.
- o **R**eview – Compare it with truth.
- o **U**nmask – Reject the lie.
- o **E**xchange – Replace it with what aligns.

Every mental exchange like this seals an energy leak.

Energy Leaks: Where Vitality Escapes

We lose energy not only through physical exhaustion but through invisible drains. These "energy leaks" often hide in plain sight—habits, relationships, or thought loops that siphon our strength.

I became aware of energy leaks during a season when I couldn't understand why I was so tired despite doing "everything right." I was eating well, resting when I could, and trying to stay grounded—yet my energy kept draining. What finally became clear was that the exhaustion wasn't physical; it was relational and emotional. I was spending enormous energy managing dynamics that weren't mine to fix—replaying conversations, anticipating reactions, staying available long past my capacity. Especially within my family, I had mistaken constant engagement for love. Once I began naming where my energy was quietly bleeding, I realized healing didn't require more effort—it required fewer leaks.

Here are common examples:

- o Chronic overcommitment — saying yes when the body says no.
- o Unresolved emotional loops — replaying conversations or regrets.
- o Toxic consumption — doom-scrolling, gossip, or negative media.

- Unexpressed creativity — suppressing the soul's natural output.
- Clutter — physical or digital disorganization that creates cognitive noise.

Each leak fragments focus and depletes your vitality. The remedy is gentle awareness, not harsh correction. Ask yourself weekly: Where is my energy leaking? What boundary or belief could seal it?

Even one sealed leak—such as reducing nightly screen time or resolving a long-avoided conversation—can restore remarkable vitality.

Energy conservation isn't withdrawal; it's wise stewardship.

Emotional Energy and the Law of Flow

I learned the law of emotional flow during a season when I was trying to stay composed while carrying more grief and betrayal than I had language for. I told myself I was being strong by holding it together, but my body told a different story—tight muscles, low energy, a constant edge of irritability. What I eventually realized was that my emotions weren't the problem; my suppression was. When I allowed myself to cry, to write honestly, to pray without editing my feelings, the stagnation began to lift. Expression didn't make me weaker—it returned circulation to places that had gone numb.

Emotion literally means energy in motion. When we repress our emotions, we interrupt the flow. Over time, that stagnation manifests as fatigue, muscle tension, or irritability. The cure is expression, not repression.

Healthy outlets—writing, prayer, music, tears, laughter—keep the current moving. The nervous system doesn't require constant positivity; it requires authenticity. When emotion moves freely, peace follows naturally.

In community settings, shared vulnerability amplifies energy instead of depleting it. This is the beauty of group healing: one person's breakthrough becomes another's permission slip. We energize one another by embodying freedom.

Spiritual Energy: The Breath of Alignment

Every faith tradition speaks of divine energy—Spirit, Ruach, Chi, Prana, Breath. This is the animating force that moves through all creation. Spiritual energy is not mystical performance; it's relational presence. When we align our breath with the Creator's rhythm, vitality flows effortlessly.

In Hebrew thought, breath and spirit share the same root. When we breathe with awareness, we remember that life itself is sustained by GOD. Each inhale invites life in; each exhale releases what we no longer need. Even breathing becomes an act of reverence.

I came to understand spiritual energy through breath in a season when my body felt perpetually braced. Conversations left me tight. Decisions felt heavy. Even prayer carried effort. What I noticed first wasn't a lack of faith, but a lack of ease in my breathing. I was inhaling shallowly, holding tension through my exhale, living as though I had to sustain myself. Learning to return to conscious breath—slow, intentional, unforced—became a turning point. With each breath, I felt myself remember that life was not something I had to manufacture. It was already being given.

When you feel drained, don't ask, "How do I get more energy?"

Ask, "Where am I disconnected from Source?" Reconnection is restoration.

Rest: The Hidden Generator

Ironically, most people try to create energy by doing more when the secret is in doing less. Rest isn't the absence of productivity—it's the foundation of it.

I used to treat rest as a reward for endurance. If everything was handled, everyone else was okay, and nothing urgent remained, *then* I could rest. That posture kept my body in a constant state of low-grade vigilance, even when I was technically "off." During seasons of emotional strain and decision fatigue, I noticed that no amount of good nutrition or movement could compensate for how unrested my nervous system felt. What finally shifted things was recognizing that rest wasn't something I earned—it was something I required in order to function with clarity and compassion. When I began honoring rest intentionally, my body responded with steadiness instead of collapse.

During deep rest, the body detoxifies, the mind consolidates memory, and the spirit receives direction. Inadequate rest interrupts the circadian rhythm, the internal clock that regulates hormonal and cellular repair. When this rhythm falters, even good nutrition and exercise can't compensate.

Practical ways to honor rest:

1. Keep a consistent bedtime and wake time.
2. Dim lights an hour before bed to cue melatonin release.
3. Avoid digital stimulation before sleep.
4. Practice a "Sabbath Pause" weekly—24 hours without agenda or devices.

As Dr. Alan Goldhammer teaches, healing is not about adding more—it's about removing interference. Rest removes interference, allowing energy to do what it was designed to do: renew.

The Flow State: Grace and Focus Combined

Psychologist Mihaly Csikszentmihalyi coined the term flow state to describe the sense of effortless immersion that occurs when skill meets challenge in harmony. In spiritual language, this is divine alignment—the moment you feel "carried" rather than controlling.

Flow arises naturally when we're rooted, intentional, and strong. You don't chase it; you create conditions for it. Safety calms the nervous system, clarity focuses attention, surrender releases resistance—and then, energy flows.

I recognized the flow state only after long seasons where it was absent. There were years when everything felt like it took a lot of effort—thinking, deciding, creating—because my energy was split between staying vigilant and staying functional. After the relational ruptures, boundary work, and surrender you've read about, something unexpected happened. There were moments when writing flowed without force, conversations unfolded without rehearsal, and decisions emerged without internal debate. I wasn't trying harder; I was resisting less. For the first time, I felt carried rather than braced. That contrast taught me what flow truly is—not intensity, but alignment.

In this state, time softens, creativity expands, and exhaustion vanishes. You are not forcing; you are being. That is the essence of Energized living.

Micro-Practice: The Daily Energy Audit

To maintain alignment, check in with your energy, just as you would with the fuel level in your car. The Daily Energy Audit is a five-minute reflection practice:

1.   Morning Scan: Before rising, ask, "How does my energy feel today—full, fragile, scattered, or steady?"
2.   Midday Reset: Step outside, breathe, and notice what activities are energizing or draining.
3.   Evening Review: Reflect on where your energy leaked and where it flowed. Offer gratitude for what sustained you.
4.   Track patterns for a week. You'll begin to see what truly fuels you. Often, it's not more sleep or supplements—it's alignment between values and actions.

Creating Energetic Boundaries

I learned the necessity of energetic boundaries when emotional boundaries alone weren't enough. Even after I limited contact and clarified expectations—particularly with my sister—I noticed my energy was still being drained. I carried conversations in my body long after they ended. I replayed words, anticipated reactions, and felt responsible for emotions that were not mine to manage.

What I realized was that while I had set relational limits, I was still *energetically overextending*. My body remained on call. Creating energetic boundaries became the next layer of healing—not withdrawing love, but reclaiming my life-force.

Just as emotional boundaries protect your peace, energetic boundaries preserve your vitality. They define where your responsibility for another's energy ends. Without them, empathy turns into exhaustion.

Simple tools for energetic hygiene:

o   Visualize returning borrowed energy to others after intense interactions.

- Limit exposure to environments that consistently leave you depleted.
- Recenter after helping others by engaging in grounding rituals (washing hands, stretching, stepping outdoors).

This isn't selfish; it's sacred maintenance. You can't pour from an empty vessel.

Energized Living and Purpose

Energy naturally rises when life aligns with purpose. Passion is not something you manufacture; it's what emerges when your values and actions intertwine. Fatigue often signals dissonance, not deficiency.

Ask yourself: "Where am I investing energy that doesn't reflect my purpose?"

Then redirect gently. Each minor course correction restores enthusiasm. Alignment rekindles fire without burnout.

In RISE, purpose isn't performance; it's presence. It's about bringing your whole self into whatever you're doing—washing dishes, teaching, creating, or parenting—with the awareness that every act can carry meaning.

Healing Energy and Service

I didn't always understand that healing energy is meant to circulate, not be consumed. For a long time, I tried to serve while still leaking—offering calm. At the same time, my own system was unsettled, giving presence while carrying unresolved pain, especially in family relationships that required far more from me than they returned. When I finally stopped over-giving and allowed my own healing to take precedence, something changed. My energy no longer felt strained or performative. It became steady. What I offered others came from fullness, not effort. Service stopped costing me myself.

When energy flows freely through one life, it spills into others. An aligned person becomes a source of calm in chaotic spaces. Your peace is contagious, and your vitality becomes testimony.

I've witnessed this countless times in my RISE Circle—when one member embodies flow, everyone breathes easier. The nervous systems of the group entrain to that steady rhythm. This is how community becomes medicine.

We don't heal for others; we heal with them. Alignment is the invitation that reminds others that they, too, can live in connection with Source.

To live energized is to live aligned—with nature's rhythm, with your body's design, with divine flow. Energy is never something you chase; it's something you allow.

When the soil is rooted, the choices are intentional, and the strength surrendered, life's current finds you. You don't have to manufacture vitality—it's what rises naturally when you are finally, fully, in tune.

That's the promise of RISE:

> Rooted in truth.
>
> Intentional in action.
>
> Strong through grace.
>
> Energized by alignment.

A Blessing for Energized Living

May your energy flow like a river—steady, clear, and alive.

May what drains you lose its hold, and what fills you multiply.

May your movement be joyful, your nourishment mindful, your thoughts light-bearing.

And may every breath remind you that life moves best through the one who surrenders to its rhythm.

Reflection Prompt

Where are my greatest energy leaks—and what truth or boundary could seal them?

Write freely, without judgment. List every small habit, belief, or relationship that drains you. Then circle the one that feels most within your power to change this week. Begin there.

PART IV

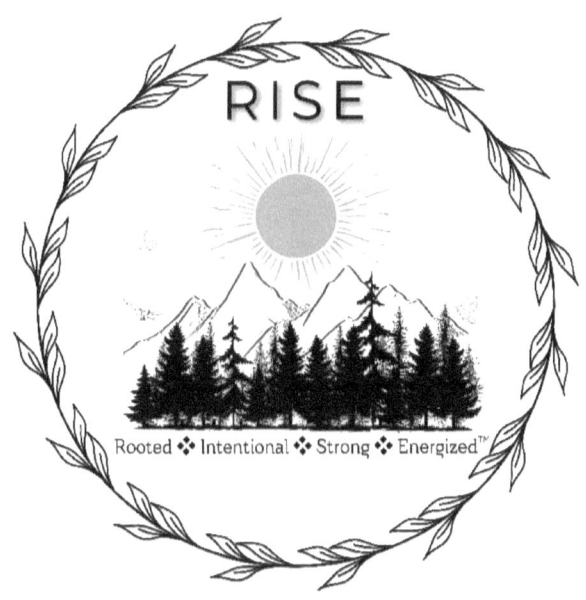

The Rhythm of Renewal

Life moves in circles, not straight lines. Every dawn becomes dusk, every inhale turns exhale, every season of growth yields to rest. The Creator designed cycles into all living things—from the heartbeat to the tides, from circadian rhythms to the sabbatical rhythm of the land. When we live against these patterns, we exhaust ourselves. When we return to them, we rediscover peace.

The RISE Circle was born from that truth. It's not a rigid system, but a gentle rhythm—a way of remembering that wholeness requires motion. Rooted, Intentional, Strong, and Energized are not separate goals but interdependent movements in the same song. They represent the flow of being: grounding, choosing, enduring, and renewing.

In this circular way of living, wellness ceases to be an achievement and becomes an integral part of an ecosystem. Every part affects the others: when thought aligns, emotion settles; when emotion settles, energy flows; when energy flows, the body heals; when the body heals, the mind grows clear. The circle is not perfection—it's participation in life's ongoing balance.

Science confirms what Spirit has always whispered: human biology is rhythmic. Our circadian clock governs sleep and wakefulness, while our ultradian cycles manage focus and rest. Our hormonal patterns ebb and flow in response to the rhythms of moonlight and sunlight. To ignore these rhythms is to live disconnected from our design.

The RISE rhythm re-teaches that balance is not static—it's dynamic. Like a dancer adjusting mid-step, life's harmony emerges through micro-corrections, gentle awareness, and continuous renewal. It is never too late to step back into rhythm. Every breath, every pause, every act of self-kindness is an entry point. This is the rhythm of renewal—the sacred remembering that life is a circle, and every moment is another chance to begin again.

Chapter 15 — The Circle of Balance

When I first drew the RISE circle, it wasn't just a diagram—it was a revelation. I saw how everything I had learned through years of healing and teaching formed a complete cycle: Mind, Body, Emotion, and Energy. Each quadrant represented one aspect of being human, yet none existed alone. Balance was not about keeping them equal but allowing them to communicate.

The RISE Circle is more than a visual model—it's a mirror of life itself. Its shape reminds us that every beginning leads back to belonging.

The RISE Circle: A Living Blueprint

Picture a circle divided into four equal quadrants:

- o Mind — clarity, beliefs, focus.
- o Body — nourishment, rest, movement.
- o Emotion — empathy, self-regulation, connection.

o Energy — vitality, flow, purpose.

At the center lies Spirit—the invisible current that holds everything together.

This model isn't meant to fragment who you are but to show how intimately everything interacts. Each quadrant depends on the others, like seasons in sequence. You can't separate spring from summer or emotion from energy. They coexist and cycle endlessly.

When we neglect one, imbalance ripples through all.

How Imbalance Ripples Through the Whole

I learned how imbalance ripples through the whole, not by studying systems theory, but by living inside a body that kept giving me feedback I couldn't ignore. There were seasons when my mind spun with worry and comparison, and I felt it immediately in my body—tight shoulders, shallow breath, exhaustion that sleep didn't fix. Other times, grief and relational strain left me undernourished and unrested, and suddenly my patience thinned, my thinking fogged, and even my spiritual practices felt distant. I tried addressing each issue in isolation—fix the food, fix the thoughts, fix the schedule—but nothing held until I understood the pattern. Everything was connected. When one part of me was neglected, the rest compensated until it couldn't anymore.

If the mind becomes cluttered with worry or comparison, the body tenses, the emotions flood, and energy drains. If the body is undernourished or sleep-deprived, the mind fogs, patience shrinks, and even faith feels far away. If emotions are repressed, muscles hold tension, thoughts spiral, and fatigue ensues. If energy leaks out due to overcommitment or distraction, focus fades, digestion falters, and creativity dries up.

The circle reveals that no single area can be healed in isolation. It must be approached holistically—much like tuning an instrument rather than fixing a specific part.

Healing begins with awareness: noticing which part of the circle is calling for care today. Sometimes it's the body whispering for rest. Sometimes it's the mind asking for silence. Sometimes it's the heart longing for forgiveness. Sometimes, it's the spirit that craves connection.

Balance is found not in uniformity but in responsiveness.

Mind: The Inner Climate of Thought

There are days when you wake up already bracing—your mind running ahead of your body, replaying conversations, scanning for what needs to be fixed or avoided. You haven't done anything yet, but you're already tired. Your thoughts feel rushed, sharp, relentless. You notice it in your shoulders first, then in your breath. By the time you reach for your phone or start your day, the tone has already been set from the inside.

That's the moment you begin to realize how powerful the mind really is. Not as an abstract concept, but as a lived climate—one that shapes how you feel in your body, how patient you are with others, how much energy you have to give. When the mind is crowded, everything downstream feels strained. When it's tended with care, the rest of the circle softens.

The mind is the gardener of perception. Its thoughts seed every other quadrant. What we think determines what we feel, how we move, and how we use energy. That's why mental hygiene matters as much as physical hygiene.

Intentional thought creates coherence; unchecked thought creates chaos. When mental patterns become harsh or hurried, energy fractures. The antidote is mindfulness—slowing down enough to observe thought without attachment. Journaling, meditation, and Scripture reflection cultivate this clarity.

A practical tool: write one grounding statement each morning, such as, "Today, my thoughts will serve peace, not pressure." Revisit it when distraction or self-criticism arises. The mind's renewal sets the circle's tone.

Body: The Grounded Home

There are moments when you realize you've been living *above* your body instead of inside it. You notice it when hunger goes ignored, when fatigue is overridden, when tension becomes so familiar you stop registering it as a signal. Your body has been speaking for a long time—through tight jaws, shallow breath, restless sleep—but you've learned to translate those messages as inconvenience rather than information. Coming back into the body doesn't happen all at once. It begins with listening, by noticing what feels braced and what feels eased. Remember that you don't live *around* your body— you live *within* it.

The body is the circle's vessel—the soil through which everything grows. It keeps the score of imbalances and the memory of peace. Our society often treats the body as either an idol or an afterthought; however, true balance sees it as a sacred instrument.

To care for the body is to honor the Creator's design. It doesn't require perfection—just partnership. Feed it foods that come from the ground, water that flows, and air that moves. Rest when weary. Stretch when stiff. Touch the earth. Let sunlight kiss your skin.

These small acts of embodied respect generate enormous energetic return.

When the body feels safe and nourished, emotional storms soften, and spiritual clarity deepens. The physical always grounds the metaphysical.

Emotion: The Language of the Heart

There are moments when emotion shows up before words do—tightness in the chest, a lump in the throat, a sudden wave you didn't schedule. You might try to reason your way through it, explain it away, or stay productive enough to outrun it. But emotion doesn't disappear when ignored; it waits. When it's finally given attention, you realize it wasn't there to overwhelm you—it was trying to communicate. Not everything you feel needs to be fixed. Some things just need to be *heard*.

Emotion connects the inner and outer worlds. It colors thought, informs energy, and moves the body. Emotion is the bridge—the translator between logic and intuition.

Unregulated emotions distort perception, while integrated emotions deepen wisdom. Emotional balance doesn't mean neutrality; it is a state of flow. You feel fully but don't drown. Practices like breath prayer, expressive writing, or compassionate self-talk reopen emotional pathways that shame once shut.

A healthy circle feels. Tears water the roots of truth; laughter aerates the soil of joy. Emotion becomes movement rather than weight.

Energy: The Expression of Alignment

There are days when energy feels effortless—you move through tasks with clarity, your body feels responsive, and creativity comes without strain. And then there are days when everything feels heavier than it should. Not because you're doing more, but because something inside you is misaligned. You might still be functioning, still showing up, but it takes more effort than it used to. That's often the first clue. Energy doesn't disappear randomly; it responds to truth. When something inside you knows you're pushing against what's real, vitality quietly withdraws.

Energy is the circle's current—the invisible force that powers all else. It is how truth moves through form. When aligned, it feels like vitality, creativity, ease. When misaligned, it feels like fatigue, frustration, and disconnection.

Energy flows freely when thought is clear, emotions are expressed, and the body is cared for. This is why healing in one area automatically revitalizes the others. Every choice that aligns your outer life with your inner truth multiplies energy.

Conversely, resisting truth—saying yes when you mean no, pretending when you need honesty—creates leaks. Energy leaks are the silent thieves of joy. The RISE rhythm teaches us to seal those leaks gently through self-awareness and alignment.

The Biological Circle: How Science Reflects Spirit

There was a point when my body started insisting on patterns I had spent years overriding. I would crash at the same time each afternoon. My focus would come in waves instead of staying steady. Sleep felt restorative some nights and elusive on others, depending on how much I had pushed or ignored myself earlier in the day. At first, I treated these fluctuations as problems to solve. Over time, I realized they were invitations—to stop fighting the way I was made and start cooperating with it. My body wasn't malfunctioning; it was keeping rhythm.

Modern science now validates what spiritual wisdom has known for millennia: we are rhythmic beings. Our circadian rhythm governs sleep, metabolism, and hormone balance. Our ultradian cycles, which occur roughly every 90 minutes, control our focus and rest patterns. Even heart rate variability reveals the dance between tension and release.

When we live counter to these rhythms—ignoring rest, skipping meals, resisting emotion—the circle strains. But when we honor them, vitality returns. Morning light resets the clock. Evening stillness lowers cortisol. Balanced meals stabilize mood. Gentle movement restores lymphatic flow. Every biological system sings in harmony when the rhythm is respected.

The RISE circle mirrors these cycles: Rooted (rest), Intentional (focus), Strong (stretch), Energized (release). It's the physiology of faithfulness—living as creation, not competition.

The Spiritual Circle: Returning to Wholeness

There were seasons when I thought moving forward meant leaving things behind—past versions of myself, old lessons, even familiar truths. But I kept noticing something else happening. The same themes returned, not to accuse me, but to deepen me. Rest would call me back after striving. Clarity would return after confusion. Strength would be asked of me again, but this time with more softness. What once felt like repetition slowly revealed itself as refinement. I wasn't going in circles—I was being drawn inward, toward something steadier.

Spiritually, the circle is covenantal. It represents eternal return—our continual movement back toward Source. In Hebraic understanding, time itself is cyclical: feasts, Sabbaths, seasons—all designed to bring us repeatedly into alignment with divine order.

RISE invites us to live the same way: revisiting each anchor not as repetition but as refinement. Every time you move through Rooted, Intentional, Strong, and Energized, you spiral upward into deeper wholeness. The circle doesn't trap—it transforms.

The center of the circle is shalom—not just peace as calm, but peace as completion. Wholeness that touches every direction at once. To live from this center is to live from balance, even when the edges tremble.

The Circle in Practice

You can embody the RISE Circle rhythm daily:

Morning: Begin with Rooted. Ground your body and mind in gratitude. Breathe. Stretch. Pray.

Midday: Shift into Intentional. Revisit your focus. Realign your energy with purpose.

Afternoon: Embody Strong. Choose grace in tension, courage in boundaries, softness in effort.

Evening: Flow into Energized. Release what's heavy. Nourish, rest, and restore.

This daily rhythm mirrors the natural arc of the sun—rising from stillness, shining with purpose, softening through surrender, and restoring through night. The same rhythm can be applied weekly, seasonally, and even across the stages of life.

Each pass through the circle reveals new wisdom. The goal is not to stay centered perfectly, but to keep returning. The circle welcomes you again and again.

When the Circle Falters

There were times when I felt off long before I could explain why. I wasn't doing anything "wrong," yet my body felt heavy, my patience thin, my thoughts louder than usual. In the past, I would have pushed through—assuming the discomfort meant weakness or regression. What changed was learning to listen instead of explain. When I paused and asked what part of me was asking for care, the answer was often compassionate and straightforward: I needed rest, or quiet, or space to feel what I had been carrying. The circle didn't condemn me for being out of balance—it showed me where I could return.

Imbalance isn't failure—it's feedback. When you feel drained, anxious, or numb, it's simply one quadrant signaling its need for care. Pause and ask:

"Which part of my circle is asking for attention?"

> If the body aches, perhaps you've ignored rest.
>
> If the mind spins, perhaps clarity needs space.
>
> If emotion overwhelms, expression is overdue.
>
> If energy wanes, alignment needs to be restored.

This question turns guilt into guidance. The circle becomes a compass, not a cage.

Reflection and Renewal

The RISE circle invites reflection, not rigidity. Every end-of-day, week, or season, you can trace your inner rhythm by journaling:

- o Where did I feel most alive?
- o What drained me unexpectedly?
- o Which anchor felt stable, and which wobbled?
- o What truth or practice might bring balance back?

Through reflection, imbalance becomes instruction. Renewal follows naturally because awareness restores rhythm.

Living the Circle Collectively

Communities flourish when people grow together. In our RISE Circle, each gathering centers on a specific topic related to whole-being wellness: health, community, spirituality, relationships, food, emotional growth, and more. Instead of analyzing which quadrant someone is in, we reflect on shared questions. Each person takes time to listen inwardly, reflect on their current season, and speak from their lived experience.

These conversations create a rhythm of connection. One week, we explore grounding practices; another week, we discuss boundaries; another week, we focus on joy, nourishment, or rest. The reflections are personal, yet they strengthen the collective. As each person engages honestly with the topic, the group becomes a place of support, accountability, and gentle transformation.

This kind of shared reflection mirrors the way nature grows— individual roots strengthened in the presence of others. Balance doesn't happen in isolation; it deepens in community. The healthier we become within ourselves, the more wholeness we naturally bring into all the circles around us.

A Circle Without End

When we live cyclically, life stops feeling like constant loss and starts feeling like a return. Seasons no longer threaten; they teach. Endings become beginnings. Fatigue becomes an invitation, not a flaw.

You'll know you're living the rhythm of renewal when presence replaces pressure. You'll stop striving for balance and start sensing it. It won't be perfect—but it will be peaceful.

That peace, that rhythm, that returning—that is the miracle of the RISE Circle:

You don't have to find balance.

You simply have to remember it.

Reflection Prompt

Which part of my circle needs care?

Close your eyes, take three slow breaths, and scan your being—mind, body, emotion, and energy. Notice which feels most tender or tired. Write one sentence beginning, "I will care for this part of me by…" Let that intention become your act of balance for today.

Chapter 16 — The Science of Rhythm: When Biology Meets Balance

There's a rhythm to everything living.

The ocean swells and retreats. The moon waxes and wanes. Birds migrate. Trees shed and bud again. Even our cells hum to invisible cycles that govern life's timing. To be human is to live within these patterns — yet modern life has silenced much of their song.

In our 24/7 culture of artificial light, constant noise, and digital clocks, we've forgotten that the body keeps time in its own sacred way. Balance isn't just a poetic metaphor; it's a biological truth. When we honor our innate rhythms, healing becomes natural. When we fight them, fatigue, anxiety, and disease follow.

The RISE philosophy calls us back to harmony — not through control, but through cooperation with creation. This is the bridge between spirit and science: living aligned with the body's divine design.

Understanding the Body's Inner Clocks

Hidden within every cell of your body are molecular timekeepers called circadian clocks. These tiny oscillators regulate sleep, digestion, hormone release, immune defense, and even emotional tone. Together, they form your circadian rhythm — a roughly 24-hour cycle responding to light, food, temperature, and activity.

At the center of it all sits the suprachiasmatic nucleus (SCN) — a cluster of neurons in the hypothalamus that synchronizes your internal clocks. The SCN receives direct signals from the eyes, translating sunlight into a cellular rhythm. Every morning, light entering the retina tells the brain, "It's time to wake, to produce cortisol for alertness." Every evening, darkness whispers, "It's time to rest, to release melatonin for repair."

When we ignore these cues — staying up late under blue light, skipping meals, or living disconnected from nature's cycles — the entire orchestra of the body falls out of tune. The result? Fatigue, inflammation, emotional volatility, and a subtle sense of disconnection that no amount of coffee or motivation can fix.

I didn't begin honoring my body's inner clocks because I mastered the science; I began because my body stopped tolerating being ignored. When I started aligning my days with light and dark— waking with the morning, dimming the evening, eating at regular intervals, letting rest be timely instead of delayed—I noticed something subtle but profound. My moods steadied. My energy felt cleaner, less forced. Sleep became restorative instead of elusive.

What felt like discipline at first turned out to be relief. My body wasn't demanding perfection—it was asking for partnership. Listening to its timing became one of the most compassionate forms of self-respect I've ever practiced. When I stopped fighting time, my body remembered how to heal.

Beyond Circadian: The Wider Rhythms of Life

Biological time doesn't stop at 24 hours. Research now reveals multiple layers of rhythm pulsing through us:

- Circadian (daily) — ~24-hour rhythm regulating sleep/wake, metabolism, and temperature.
- Ultradian (intra-day) — 90–120-minute focus-rest cycles affecting productivity and attention.
- Circaseptan (weekly) — seven-day cycles observed in immune response, heart rate, and mood — echoing the biblical pattern of the Sabbath.
- Circannual (seasonal) — yearly shifts in hormones, appetite, mood, and even creativity, tied to light exposure and temperature changes.

Ancient traditions understood these patterns long before modern science named them. The seven-day rhythm of work and rest, the new moon celebrations, and the agricultural festivals of planting and harvest all reflected the body's deep attunement to time. Our ancestors didn't just live in nature; they lived with it. They rose with dawn, rested at dusk, and worked with the seasons — never mistaking busyness for worth. To return to rhythm is to remember we are part of creation, not apart from it.

I didn't begin noticing these wider rhythms because I was looking for them; I noticed them because my body kept responding when I honored them. There were weeks when I tried to push past natural pauses and felt my focus collapse mid-day. Seasons when forcing productivity left me depleted instead of accomplished. And moments when allowing a true Sabbath—mental, emotional, not just physical—restored more clarity than an entire week of effort. What became clear was this: my body already knew these rhythms. I had simply learned to ignore them. Returning to them didn't make life smaller—it made it saner. I stopped measuring my worth by output and started measuring it by alignment. Rhythm didn't restrict my life—it gave it back its breath.

Zeitgebers — The "Time-Givers" of the Body

In German, the word zeitgeber means "time-giver." These are the environmental cues that set our internal clocks. The main zeitgebers are:

Zeitgeber (Time-Giver)	How It Sets the Clock	Examples & Tips
Light	The most powerful synchronizer. Morning sunlight boosts cortisol, serotonin, and body temperature.	Spend 10–15 minutes in natural morning light; dim lights after sunset
Food	Meal timing influences liver and gut clocks.	Eat at consistent times; avoid late-night eating.
Movement	Physical activity signals wakefulness and regulates mood.	Move early in the day or during natural energy peaks.

Zeitgeber (Time-Giver)	How It Sets the Clock	Examples & Tips
Temperature	Cooler temps signal rest; warmer temps cue alertness.	Lower room temp at night for deeper sleep.
Social Connection	Emotional engagement synchronizes circaseptan and hormonal rhythms.	Maintain regular relational rhythms— conversation, shared meals, community time.
Rest and Silence	Recovery phases regulate parasympathetic function.	Observe daily "pauses" for prayer, breathwork, or meditation.

Each time-giver resets your internal clock toward balance. Disrupt them — through erratic schedules, constant screen light, or isolation — and rhythm unravels.

Body Systems Affected by Circadian Rhythm

System	Circadian Influence	Signs of Imbalance
Mood & Mental Health	Serotonin and dopamine fluctuate with daylight; adequate morning light stabilizes emotion.	Irritability, anxiety, depression, and brain fog.
Metabolism	Insulin sensitivity peaks in the morning; nighttime eating raises blood sugar and fat storage.	Cravings, weight gain, sluggish digestion.

System	Circadian Influence	Signs of Imbalance
Hormones	Cortisol, melatonin, thyroid, and reproductive hormones follow daily patterns.	Fatigue, insomnia, menstrual irregularity, adrenal exhaustion.
Immunity	Immune cells patrol on a circadian schedule; sleep loss suppresses defense.	Frequent colds, slow healing, and inflammation.
Cellular Repair	DNA repair and autophagy occur mainly during sleep.	Premature aging, poor recovery, low resilience.

The entire body dances to time's rhythm. To ignore the music is to trip over your own design.

The RISE Anchors Through the Lens of Rhythm

For a long time, I tried to live well by effort alone. I focused on doing the right things—eating better, thinking better, believing better—yet something still felt off. My days were uneven. Some mornings felt grounded; others felt rushed before they began. I could be disciplined for a while, then suddenly depleted without understanding why. What eventually became clear wasn't that I lacked commitment, but that I lacked rhythm. I was applying good practices out of sequence, out of season, and often against my own biology.

As I began paying attention—not just to *what* I was doing, but *when* and *how*—the RISE anchors stopped feeling like concepts and started behaving like a living cycle. Rooted wasn't just about truth; it was about anchoring my body in time. Intentional wasn't just about choice; it was about transitions. Strong wasn't about pushing;

it was about pacing. Energized wasn't something I summoned; it emerged when everything else was aligned. The anchors revealed themselves not as tasks to master, but as rhythms to return to.

Every anchor of RISE mirrors a biological phase — Rooted, Intentional, Strong, and Energized are not abstract ideas; they're cyclical expressions of natural order. When practiced in rhythm, they form a daily and lifelong pattern of vitality.

Rooted — Consistent Wake/Sleep and Sunlight Grounding

Being Rooted means honoring your anchor points in time — waking and sleeping consistently, aligning your day with the sun's rhythm.

Science:

> Melatonin production begins around 9 p.m. when light dims. Cortisol peaks 30 minutes after waking, preparing the body for action. Disrupting this pattern (through late-night light exposure or inconsistent sleep) causes hormonal confusion and emotional instability.

Practice:

- o Wake within the same 30-minute window daily, even on weekends.
- o Expose your eyes to natural light within one hour of waking.
- o Step outside barefoot or breathe fresh air — grounding reconnects electrical and energetic balance.
- o Avoid screens 1–2 hours before bed; use candlelight or dimmed lamps.

When you rise and rest with creation's rhythm, you become part of its stability. Rooted living restores your sense of belonging in time.

Intentional — Aligned Mealtimes and Mindful Transitions

Intentional living brings awareness to timing — not just what you do, but when. Each choice becomes a micro-alignment with your biological design.

Science:

> Metabolic efficiency depends on circadian cues. The digestive system functions best when meals are eaten during daylight. Nighttime eating disrupts insulin and liver rhythms. Even mental focus follows ultradian (90-minute) cycles — requiring short rests for sustained performance.

Practice:

- Eat main meals within a 10-hour window (e.g., 8 a.m.–6 p.m.).
- Transition intentionally between tasks: take three slow breaths, stretch, or hydrate before beginning something new.
- Create "light cues" in your workspace: bright during work hours, dimmer toward evening.
- Schedule prayer or reflection pauses at natural breaks to restore mental alignment.

Intention gives shape to rhythm. Without it, we drift; however, with it, we dance.

Strong — Pacing Work/Rest Cycles

Strength isn't perpetual output — it's endurance through recovery. Just as muscles grow during rest, the nervous system regenerates during pause.

Science:

> Ultradian cycles show that focus naturally declines after 90 minutes. Continuing without rest raises cortisol and lowers creativity. Heart rate variability (HRV) reveals oscillations between exertion and relaxation and defines resilience.

Practice:

- o Work in 90-minute blocks, followed by 10–20 minutes of movement or stillness.
- o Plan physical exercise in daylight hours to support the circadian wake phase.
- o Practice "Sabbath micro-rests" — moments of stillness during each day before pushing forward.
- o When fatigued, pause. Forcing through leads to burnout.

The Strong rhythm honors both tension and release — a grace-filled strength that breathes rather than breaks.

Energized — Flowing with Natural Peaks

Energized living is the art of working with your body's natural highs and lows rather than against them.

Science:

> Alertness typically rises mid-morning, dips in the early afternoon, then lifts again around early evening. Creativity often peaks when the mind relaxes — during walks, showers, or transitions. Ignoring these waves leads to frustration and inefficiency.

Practice:

- o Schedule analytical or demanding tasks for your natural energy peaks.
- o Take a short walk or nap during midafternoon dips to reset.
- o Hydrate and breathe deeply to maintain oxygen flow.
- o Avoid caffeine late in the day; let your energy wind down gracefully.

Energy is not constant—it's cyclical. To ride its rhythm is to experience flow, not fatigue.

Rhythm as Medicine

Every ancient healing system—Hebrew, Ayurvedic, Chinese, Indigenous—recognized time as medicine. The wrong remedy at the wrong time is ineffective, but the right action at the right moment restores harmony. Science now supports this:

- o Medications taken at certain times of day are more effective ("chronotherapy").
- o Eating within daylight hours improves metabolism.
- o Exercising in morning light increases sleep quality.
- o Expressing gratitude or prayer before rest lowers blood pressure and stress hormones.

Healing is not only what you do—it's when.

When you begin living this way, life stops feeling like resistance and starts feeling like resonance.

Restoring the Sabbath Rhythm

Restoring the Sabbath rhythm in our home began as a theological decision. It was a choice to trust that GOD's design was not symbolic or optional, but authoritative and life-giving. My husband, our daughter, and I chose to order our week around what Scripture had already named as holy (set apart)—not because we were rested, but because we were not.

What followed surprised us. As we consistently honored the seventh day, its effects rippled outward into our bodies, our relationships, and the atmosphere of our home. The pace slowed. Nervous systems settled. Joy returned without effort.

Even our environment seemed to adapt—our cats instinctively grew quieter and more restful on Sabbath, and even the occasional sugar ant visitors appeared to observe the pause, arriving and retreating with uncanny regularity. What began as obedience became alignment. Theology moved from belief into biology, and from biology into the environment.

Among all biological cycles, the seven-day rhythm (circaseptan) remains one of the most mysterious. Even in isolation experiments where people were cut off from sunlight and clocks, the body continued to follow a roughly seven-day oscillation in immune activity, heart rate, and emotional state. Scripture's Sabbath pattern wasn't superstition—it was synchronization.

The seventh day invites renewal not merely as religious observance but as a neurological reset. It aligns your inner clock with divine rest. Every Sabbath, your cortisol drops, serotonin stabilizes, and creativity rebounds. This is not laziness; it's liberation. In resting, you return to the rhythm of Eden — where life was meant to flow, not strive.

Practical Ways to Reclaim Rhythm

1. Morning Light Ritual: Step outside for 10 minutes of unfiltered sunlight. Let your eyes (not your phone) greet the day.
2. Consistent Mealtimes: Eat breakfast, lunch, and dinner at roughly the same times each day.
3. Midday Movement: Move your body during daylight — a brisk walk, gardening, or stretching.
4. Evening Wind-Down: Reduce blue light exposure 1–2 hours before sleep. Read, stretch, pray.
5. Weekly Sabbath: Choose one day to disconnect from digital noise and reconnect with rest. We chose the traditional Saturday, seventh day Sabbath.
6. Seasonal Awareness: Adjust sleep, food, and activity with the seasons—lighter meals in summer, deeper rest in winter.
7. Energy Check-Ins: Ask throughout the day, "Is what I'm doing matching my current energy or forcing against it?"

Each small alignment multiplies the effect. Rhythm isn't another task—it's the permission to stop fighting your own nature.

When Rhythm Heals the Nervous System

I didn't realize how deeply my nervous system needed rhythm until it finally began to relax. After years of unpredictability—relational strain, vigilance, seasons where I stayed braced even when nothing was actively wrong—my body had learned to expect disruption and traumatic drama.

What rhythm offered wasn't control, but reassurance. As our days and weeks became more predictable, as rest and Sabbath anchored time itself, something inside me softened. Sleep deepened. My reactions slowed. I no longer startled so easily inside my own life.

Rhythm didn't erase the past, but it taught my body a new present. One where safety wasn't temporary, and peace didn't have to be earned.

Trauma and chronic stress disrupt internal timing. Sleep becomes irregular, appetite blurs, emotions swing wide. Reestablishing rhythm signals safety to the body. Predictable patterns—consistent wake, meal, and rest times—retrain the nervous system to trust stability.

You are teaching your body: I am safe now. I can rest, digest, and feel.

This is why rhythm heals trauma—it restores predictability where chaos once ruled. Balance, then, isn't only physical—it's deeply psychological and spiritual. Rhythm is a form of love.

Reflection Prompt

What Rhythm Is My Body Asking Me to Honor Today?

Sit quietly and breathe.

Ask your body, "What rhythm are you asking me to remember?"

Maybe it's the need for more sleep. Perhaps it's a pause before the next project. Maybe it's an earlier sunrise walk or a digital sunset.

Listen without judgment. The body's wisdom often whispers where the mind shouts.

Write one intention in your journal that begins with:

"Today, I will honor my rhythm by…"

Then keep it small and doable. A single rhythmic shift practiced daily changes everything.

Chapter 17 — The Fourfold Rhythm of Living

There is a rhythm in all of life—a pulse that began when the Creator spoke light into being. Morning and evening. Work and rest. Growth and stillness. I didn't always know how to live inside that rhythm. Much of my early life trained me to stay alert rather than aligned, to brace rather than trust. When chaos becomes familiar, stillness can feel unsafe, and renewal feels like something you earn rather than receive.

For years, my life moved in spurts rather than cycles—long stretches of endurance followed by collapse. I mistook survival for strength and recovery for failure. Even later, when relational ruptures in adulthood—especially within my own family—forced me to confront limits I could no longer ignore, I realized how deeply I had learned to live *out of rhythm*. I could recover, but I didn't yet know how to renew.

What the RISE framework eventually revealed was not a new way to push forward, but a way to return—again and again—to a pattern older than my pain. It was never meant to be a static list of anchors, but a living cycle—one that renews the body, refreshes the mind, restores the heart, and reconnects the spirit. When I began aligning with that rhythm, life stopped feeling like constant repair. Renewal became ongoing, not occasional.

This is the essence of the Fourfold Rhythm of Living:

1. Daily Renewal

2. Weekly Renewal

3. Seasonal Renewal

4. Lifelong Renewal

Each cycle reflects both the science of chronobiology—the study of time in biology—and the sacred wisdom that time itself is holy when lived with intention. What I love most about this rhythm is its mercy. It's self-correcting. You don't have to master it or keep it perfectly. You only have to notice when you've drifted and gently return. That, too, is part of the rhythm.

1. Daily Renewal — The Rhythm of Breath and Balance

Each day is a microcosm of a lifetime.

We rise, create, rest, and begin again. The circadian rhythm — that 24-hour internal clock — governs nearly every process in the body: alertness, digestion, hormones, temperature, and mood.

When we live aligned with it, energy flows naturally. When we don't, even the best intentions feel like pushing uphill.

Daily renewal begins with three sacred anchors: breath, gratitude, and nourishment.

Breath

I learned the power of breath when my body stopped responding to reasoning. There were moments when words, logic, and even prayer felt out of reach—especially during seasons of relational stress and betrayal. My nervous system would surge before my mind could catch up. Breath became the first place I could return. I noticed that when I slowed my breathing, my body followed. My shoulders softened. My jaw unclenched. I didn't need answers; I needed presence. Breath reminded me that safety could be experienced *now*, not just hoped for later. It became my daily way of re-entering my body instead of abandoning it.

Breath is the most immediate way to reset your internal clock. A single deep breath signals the nervous system to shift from stress to safety. Slow breathing synchronizes the heart and brain, regulating emotional and physical rhythm.

Every inhale is an act of receiving; every exhale, an act of release. To breathe consciously is to remember you're alive — here, now, present.

Try this RISE Breath Rhythm:

- o   Inhale for 4 counts (receive).
- o   Hold for 2 (settle).
- o   Exhale for 6 (release).
- o   Pause for 2 (rest).

Repeat three times each morning or when you feel uncentered.

Gratitude

Gratitude didn't come naturally to me in hard seasons; it had to be practiced deliberately. There were days when gratitude felt almost defiant—choosing to name what was still good while things I loved were unraveling. But over time, I noticed something subtle: gratitude didn't deny grief; it stabilized me inside it.

When I began each morning by naming one thing I was thankful for—often something as simple as breath or light—my mind softened its grip on what was missing. Gratitude didn't fix my circumstances, but it anchored my perception. It helped me inhabit the day I was actually living, instead of the one I was mourning or fearing.

Gratitude resets your mental rhythm the same way light resets the circadian rhythm. It redirects perception toward life rather than lack.

Studies show that gratitude practices improve sleep, reduce inflammation, and stabilize serotonin levels. Spiritually, gratitude transforms daily routines into sacred rituals — turning breakfast into a blessing, work into worship, and rest into reverence.

Begin each morning with one sentence:

> "Today, I'm thankful for the breath that carries me
> and the rhythm that sustains me."

You can choose your own or use this one.

Nourishment

My relationship with nourishment shifted when I stopped treating food as fuel to optimize and started treating it as communication. During periods of stress, I could immediately feel when meals were skipped, delayed, or eaten without presence—my blood sugar climbed, my patience thinned, my sleep fractured. Choosing to eat regularly and simply became an act of regulation, not control. I learned that nourishment wasn't about eating "perfectly" or anything fancy, but it was about cooperating with my body's need for consistency. Each meal became a way of saying, *I'm listening. I'm here. You matter.*

What you eat — and when — sets your metabolic rhythm. Eating with the sun (breakfast and lunch as main meals, lighter dinner) mirrors your body's energy curve. Skipping meals or eating late confuses the liver and pancreas, disrupting blood sugar and sleep.

Nourish regularly and mindfully, not as performance but as a participation in creation.

Daily renewal is not a to-do list — it's a rhythm of being.

It's how you begin and end each day with awareness, letting small moments keep you aligned with the greater flow.

2. Weekly Renewal — The Rhythm of Rest and Relationship

For much of my life, weeks blurred together. I measured time by what needed to be done, not by what needed to be restored. Even after I began caring for my body and mind more intentionally, something still felt incomplete until we reclaimed a true weekly pause in our home.

When my husband, our daughter, and I reordered our lives around Sabbath—not as an idea, but as a fixed point in time—everything slowed in a way that effort never achieved. The pause became a teacher. It exposed how often I equated usefulness with worth and how deeply my nervous system had been trained to stay "on."

Weekly renewal didn't make life smaller; it made it more spacious. And relationships had room to breathe again.

While daily rhythm sustains the body, weekly rhythm restores the soul. Science calls it the circaseptan rhythm — a seven-day biological cycle regulating immune function, heart rate, and emotional equilibrium. Scripture calls it Sabbath — a sacred pause built into the pattern of creation itself.

Both point to the same truth: humans are not machines designed for endless motion.

We are rhythmic beings who require cycles of exertion *and* restoration.

The Sacred Pause

What surprised me most about Sabbath was not how much stopped, but how much returned. Laughter came back. Curiosity came back. Sabbath taught me that rest is not inactivity—it's trust embodied in time. Choosing to stop once a week retrained my body to believe that provision didn't depend on my constant effort. The pause became the pulse that reminded me who I was before productivity named me.

The Sabbath rhythm is more than a religious observance — it's a design principle. Rest is not a reward for work; it's part of the work. Each week, we are invited to stop striving and remember that our worth is not tied to our output.

Neuroscience confirms what ancient wisdom has long known: downtime improves problem-solving, enhances creativity, and strengthens memory. Physically, cortisol (the stress hormone) drops after 24 hours of rest, allowing the body to heal and rebalance.

Spiritually, Sabbath recenters us in trust — reminding us that life continues even when we stop trying to control it.

You might practice Sabbath in different ways:

- o Silence — turn off notifications, step away from screens.
- o Slowness — cook, walk, or visit the garden without rush.
- o Stillness — rest, nap, or simply breathe.
- o Sanctuary — gather with family or community for shared gratitude.

Weekly renewal isn't about escaping life; it's about reentering it restored. The pause is the pulse of presence.

Community as Restoration

I learned the restorative power of community most clearly after relational fractures in my own family. When familiar bonds felt unstable, gathering with others who practiced presence became a lifeline. Sabbath gatherings, RISE circles, shared meals, and weekly touchpoints didn't replace what was lost, but they regulated what remained. Community reminded my nervous system that safety could exist beyond one relationship. Healing didn't happen in isolation—it happened in rhythm with others who were also learning how to rest, listen, and return.

Social connection acts as a biological regulator — oxytocin, serotonin, and immune cells all respond positively to belonging. This is why isolation depletes while togetherness renews.

Gathering weekly — in worship, shared meals, or RISE circles — stabilizes both body and mind. The collective rhythm amplifies individual renewal. Weekly rhythm is where personal wellness becomes communal wholeness.

3. Seasonal Renewal — The Rhythm of Nature's Transitions

There was a time when I expected myself to function the same way year-round—to produce, engage, and endure regardless of season. Ignoring seasonal shifts felt normal until my body began to resist them. Energy waxed and waned. Creativity came in waves. Grief surfaced more readily in certain months. Once I stopped interpreting these changes as inconsistency and began reading them as seasonal intelligence, something softened. Nature wasn't failing to be constant; it was being faithful to change. I realized I was allowed to do the same.

If the daily rhythm aligns you with light and the weekly rhythm restores your spirit, then the seasonal rhythm teaches adaptability. Life changes, and so must your habits. The body, like the earth, moves through seasons of growth, stillness, shedding, and bloom.

Chronobiology shows that the length of daylight, temperature, and humidity affect hormone production, appetite, and mood. The more we mirror these external patterns, the more balanced we feel internally.

Spring — Renewal and Reawakening

Spring has always felt like permission to hope again. After long winters—both literal and emotional—it marked the return of curiosity, gentle optimism, and growth. In seasons following loss or strain, spring didn't erase what had happened, but it invited me to plant again without certainty. I learned to start small: a new habit, a cleared surface, a quiet intention. Spring taught me that beginnings don't have to be loud to be real.

Spring invites detoxification and new beginnings. Light increases, metabolism quickens, and creativity rises.

Spiritually, it's a time for planting seeds — both literal and symbolic.

Focus on fresh foods, morning movement, and new intentions.

Practice: Rise earlier with the sun; write a new affirmation; clean a space in your home to welcome clarity.

Summer — Expansion and Expression

Summer revealed to me how much joy requires space. When life allowed for longer days, shared meals, and unhurried movement, my nervous system responded with openness. I noticed how laughter restored energy faster than discipline ever had. Summer reminded me that expression is not frivolous—it's vital. Play is not the opposite of seriousness; it's the soil where resilience grows.

Summer's long days awaken extroversion and energy. It's the season for expression, laughter, and movement.

Your circadian rhythm thrives on morning light and hydration.

Spiritually, summer asks: How am I shining?

Practice: Move outdoors, share meals with others, and savor creative play.

Autumn — Release and Reflection

Autumn became my teacher in letting go. During seasons when relationships changed, and expectations fell away, I learned that release was not loss—it was preparation. Simplifying commitments, eating grounding foods, and allowing reflection gave grief a place to land instead of leaking. Autumn taught me that holding on too tightly makes winter harsher. Letting go, done gently, makes rest possible.

Autumn teaches letting go. Trees drop leaves to prepare for rest; so must we release what's heavy.

Digestion slows, introspection deepens, and emotions surface.

Spiritually, autumn says: What am I ready to release to stay rooted in truth?

Practice: Simplify commitments, eat grounding foods (squash, lentils, root vegetables), and journal what you're ready to release.

Winter — Rest and Restoration

Winter used to feel like something to endure. Now, I recognize it as a necessary descent. In quieter months, when energy naturally turns inward, I learned to stop demanding productivity from myself. Stillness became spacious instead of empty. Prayer deepened. Rest stopped feeling like retreat and began to feel like incubation. Winter taught me that nothing is wasted when it's resting.

Winter is not death — it's incubation. The earth rests beneath silence, storing strength for what's next.

In this quiet, you recover vitality.

Sleep longer, eat warm meals, move gently, and pray deeply. This is the season for stillness and spiritual recalibration.

Practice: Light candles, read reflective works, limit external noise, and let rest do its job.

Living seasonally teaches flexibility and faith — trusting that dormancy and growth are equally sacred.

4. Lifelong Renewal — The Rhythm of Becoming

Looking back, my life has unfolded in spirals rather than straight lines. There have been seasons of building, seasons of breaking, seasons of waiting, and seasons of blooming—often repeating in new forms. What once felt like regression revealed itself as refinement. Each return carried more awareness. Lifelong renewal taught me that becoming isn't about arriving; it's about consenting to change without abandoning yourself along the way.

If daily, weekly, and seasonal rhythms align you with time, then lifelong renewal aligns you with purpose.

This is the longest rhythm — the great spiral of your becoming.

Across decades, you'll experience many "mini-seasons": times of building, times of breaking, times of stillness, times of blooming.

Each has a lesson.

Each is necessary.

When we resist change, we suffer. When we honor life's rhythm, we grow in grace.

Purpose as Pulse

I once believed purpose was something I had to define early and defend relentlessly. Experience taught me otherwise. Purpose revealed itself through listening—especially during seasons when plans fell apart. As I stayed rooted in identity rather than outcome, direction emerged organically. Purpose stopped feeling like pressure and started feeling like participation.

Your life purpose isn't a fixed destination; it's a pulse that evolves with your seasons.

When you're rooted in identity and intentional in action, purpose unfolds naturally.

Like a tree, it deepens with age — drawing from both light and shadow.

The key is curiosity. Keep asking, "What is life teaching me now?" Renewal happens when learning never stops.

Evolution Through Alignment

Each time I fell out of rhythm—through overgiving, overworking, or overexplaining—my body gave me feedback. Each return taught me something new about alignment. Growth didn't come from forcing change, but from cooperating with truth as it unfolded. Alignment became an evolution practiced gently.

Psychologists call this self-actualization. Scripture calls it transformation. Both describe the same movement — from survival to service, from doing to being.

Each time you fall out of rhythm and find your way back, you evolve.

Life becomes less about control and more about cooperation with divine design.

Legacy as the Final Renewal

Legacy became clearer to me when I realized it wasn't something I would someday leave—it was something I was already living. The way I rested, spoke, forgave, and returned set a tone others could feel. Legacy wasn't performance; it was resonance. What continues isn't what we achieve, but what we embody.

The final rhythm of legacy is not what you leave behind, but what you leave alive. It's the energy that continues to ripple through others long after you've spoken your last word.

When your life has moved in rhythm — with grace, intention, strength, and energy — your legacy becomes a living blessing. Lifelong renewal isn't about staying young; it's about staying aligned. The rhythm of your life becomes a song others can follow.

Integrating Science and Sacred Rhythm

Modern science calls it chronobiology. Ancient faith calls it sacred rhythm. Both describe the same truth: health and holiness flow from harmony with time.

The more I studied science, the more reverent I became. Chronobiology didn't replace faith—it confirmed it. What Scripture named as wisdom, the body experienced as safety. Rhythm became the meeting place between cells and spirit, biology and belief. Living in rhythm felt less like discipline and more like belonging.

When you rise with light, rest with dark, honor the week's pause, and live with the seasons, your biology begins to worship. Cells fire in praise, hormones balance in prayer, and the nervous system sings of safety.

The Hebrew word shalom means peace, but also wholeness — everything in right relationship. Living in rhythm is living in shalom.

RISE doesn't just restore balance; it teaches belonging — to time, to creation, to yourself.

Practice: Map Your RISE Rhythm

To embody this chapter, take one evening this week to create your personal rhythm map.

Divide a page into four sections:

Cycle	What Renewal Looks Like for Me	RISE Focus	Small Next Step
Daily	_____	Rooted	_____
Weekly	_____	Intentional	_____
Seasonal	_____	Strong	_____
Lifelong	_____	Energized	_____

Write what renewal means for each. Then circle the one area that feels most out of rhythm and make one small change this week.

Maybe it's setting a bedtime alarm.

Maybe it's turning your phone off on Sunday.

Maybe it's walking outside every morning for light.

Or maybe it's forgiving yourself for seasons when you forgot the song.

Rhythm doesn't demand perfection — only participation.

You don't have to master time. You only have to move with it.

Reflection Prompt

"Where am I in my rhythm right now — beginning, building, resting, or renewing?"

Whichever season you're in, it belongs.

The body, mind, and spirit were created to flow in cycles — not to burn out trying to stay in one season forever.

When you live the Fourfold Rhythm of Living, balance stops being a goal and becomes a way of being.

You live Rooted in truth, Intentional in action, Strong in grace, and Energized in flow — every day, week, season, and lifetime.

That is RISE:

> a framework, a philosophy,
>
> > and a way to remember the music of being whole.

PART V

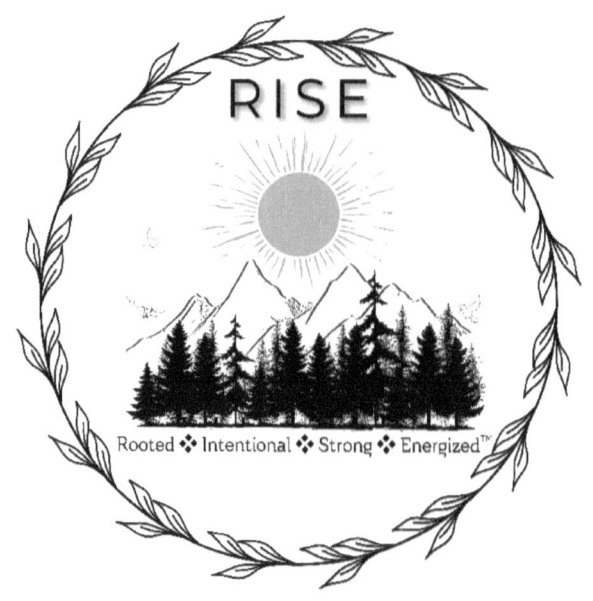

Embodiment & Community

Knowledge alone doesn't heal; embodiment does.

You can read, understand, and even believe in wellness, but until it moves through your body, transformation remains incomplete.

The body is not the bystander of your healing—it's the canvas. Every emotion leaves an impression, every belief a pattern, every breath a message. True wholeness cannot stay abstract; it must become incarnate.

The RISE philosophy was always meant to end where it began: in the body. Because once healing lives there, it starts to shape culture. When one person lives a balanced life, they influence everyone around them. Homes soften. Workplaces calm. Communities heal.

This is how movements begin—not with mass marketing, but with embodied examples. When someone walks into a room, anchored, peaceful, and present, others feel it. The nervous systems around them regulate. Energy entrains. The atmosphere shifts.

Embodiment is not about perfection; it's about integration. It's remembering that posture can preach, that breath can pray, and that presence can restore what words never could.

In this section, we move from philosophy to physiology, from concepts to culture. Because when wholeness lives in your body, it multiplies—one breath, one step, one life at a time.

Chapter 18 — The Body Remembers What the Mind Forgets

Before I ever understood embodiment, my body was already telling the story. It told it in shallow breaths I didn't notice I was holding, in shoulders that stayed lifted long after the threat had passed, in a pace that suggested urgency even when nothing was wrong. I learned early how to leave my body—to stay alert, capable, composed. It kept me functioning, but it didn't keep me whole. Long before my mind had language for trauma, betrayal, or grief, my body had already memorized them. Healing didn't begin when I understood my story. It began when I stopped arguing with what my body already knew.

The body is an autobiography written in muscle, breath, and bone.

Even when memory fades, the body remembers.

It carries what the mind cannot — every sorrow and every celebration. Every moment of joy, safety, fear, or shame has been recorded somewhere in you: in the curve of your shoulders, the depth of your breath, the rhythm of your walk. The body doesn't lie—it tells the truth of our lived experience. That truth becomes the gateway to healing.

Embodiment is not a buzzword; it's a biological necessity. You can't think your way into balance—you must feel your way there.

Somatic Integration: How Posture, Breath, and Pace Carry Beliefs

Somatic comes from the Greek sōma, meaning body.

In science and medicine, somatic refers to anything related to the physical body, especially the body as distinguished from the mind or spirit.

Somatic integration is the process of uniting your intellectual understanding of healing with your physical experience of safety and peace. It's when what you know in your head starts to show up in how you move through the world.

Posture

For years, my posture reflected vigilance rather than confidence. I didn't notice it until I began paying attention to how my body entered rooms—slightly guarded, slightly forward, always prepared. Even in moments of safety, my body stayed on guard. Learning to stand upright wasn't about looking strong; it was about letting my body know it no longer had to brace. The first time I consciously softened my shoulders and lifted my chest, I felt unexpectedly emotional. My body wasn't resisting change—it was recognizing relief.

Posture is language. Body language is a well-researched area across psychology, communication, and neuroscience. Posture is a form of body communication and is studied extensively in fields such as nonverbal communication and kinesics. A slumped spine whispers defeat. A lifted chest proclaims confidence. But more than that, it also rewires emotion. Research in psychophysiology shows that changing your posture can shift your mood within minutes.

When you sit or stand upright, you signal your nervous system that you are safe. Shoulders back, chin relaxed, breath open—these simple cues calm the body and clarify the mind.

Practice:

Pause right now. Drop your shoulders. Relax your jaw. Lengthen your spine.

Notice how your breath immediately deepens. Your body just told your brain, "You are safe."

Posture isn't only about presentation—it's about permission. You're giving your body permission to stop guarding and start receiving.

Breath

Breath became my refuge when words failed. In moments of relational rupture—especially when truth was questioned or trust was broken—my mind raced for explanation while my body tightened. I learned that slowing my breath could reach places reassurance never could. Each long exhale felt like telling my body, *You don't have to protect me right now.*

Over time, breath stopped being an exercise and became a language. It was how I learned to say yes to life again without forcing myself to feel safe before I actually did.

Breath is the bridge between body and belief. Shallow breathing often accompanies self-protection—an unconscious bracing against life. Deep breathing, by contrast, invites trust.

Trauma, grief, and chronic stress all constrict the diaphragm. Over time, this teaches the body to live in survival mode, ready for danger even in safety. Relearning to breathe fully restores the rhythm of renewal you were designed for.

Breathwork activates the vagus nerve—the body's built-in peacekeeper—shifting the nervous system from fight or flight to rest and digest. Slow exhalations cue safety more effectively than logic ever could.

Each breath becomes a physical "yes" to life again.

Pace

There was a season when my speed didn't match my surroundings. I moved quickly even in quiet spaces, ate fast even when I wasn't hungry, spoke efficiently when tenderness was needed. Slowing down felt uncomfortable at first, almost irresponsible. But when I practiced moving more slowly—especially during walks—I noticed something profound: my thoughts softened. My body stopped scanning. Presence returned not because I demanded it, but because I finally gave it time to arrive.

The pace of your movement reflects the pace of your mind. In seasons of imbalance, we rush—walking fast, talking fast, eating fast, thinking fast. But when you slow your pace intentionally, the body tells the mind: There's no emergency.

Walking slowly, eating slowly, or even speaking with pauses is somatic grace in motion.

Try this: walk one minute slower than usual. Notice how your awareness widens. You begin to see colors, hear birds, and feel the air. That's what presence feels like—it's pace in alignment with peace.

The Nervous System as a Map of Memory

Understanding that the nervous system carries memory reframed my entire healing journey. It helped me release the shame of "knowing better" but still reacting. My body wasn't betraying my progress; it was protecting me based on old information. When I stopped treating my reactions as failures and started treating them as messages, compassion replaced frustration. The body doesn't need to be corrected into safety—it needs to experience it.

The nervous system records your history. Every shock, every delight, every disappointment leaves a trace. Over time, these traces shape how your body reacts to new experiences.

If your past taught you that rest was unsafe or that stillness was lazy, your body may resist slowing down even when your mind knows better.

If love once hurt, your body may brace at intimacy even while your heart longs for connection. This is why awareness alone isn't enough—your body must experience new safety to believe it. Somatic integration provides that experience. It helps you replace the reflexes of survival with the rhythms of shalom.

The good news? The body is incredibly forgiving. The moment it feels safe, it starts to heal.

Embodiment as Truth-Telling Through Movement and Presence

There were times when my body told the truth long before my voice could. Tears arrived before words. Fatigue showed up before boundaries did. My body knew when something was misaligned, even when I tried to reason it out. Learning to trust embodiment meant letting my physical responses serve as data rather than distractions. When I stopped silencing my body, my mind no longer had to work so hard to defend what wasn't true.

Embodiment is honesty made visible. It's when your outer life begins to express your inner truth. When you're rooted, your body moves with gravity rather than against it. When you're intentional, your gestures become deliberate and meaningful. When you're strong, your boundaries are evident in your posture and tone. When you're energized, your presence radiates vitality that others can feel.

This is why embodiment is contagious—peace spreads through nervous system resonance. The same way a tuning fork vibrates in sympathy with another, your calm body teaches others to calm.

> Your body becomes a sermon of safety.
>
> Your stillness becomes an invitation.
>
> Your alignment becomes ministry.

Embodiment is also emotional honesty. Tears are truth in liquid form. Shaking hands may be truth exiting through the body. Laughter is truth released through joy. Movement—dance, walking, stretching—becomes a kind of prayer where the body preaches what words can't.

When your body tells the truth, the mind no longer has to defend it.

Practice: Body-Scan Meditation

This simple practice helps the body and mind reconnect. It's both science and sacred ritual — lowering cortisol, increasing interoception (body awareness), and calming emotional reactivity.

Step 1: Set the Environment

Find a quiet space. Sit or lie down comfortably. Let your hands rest loosely. Close your eyes if it's safe to do so.

Step 2: Ground in Breath

Take three deep breaths. Inhale through the nose for four counts, exhale through the mouth for six. With each exhale, feel the weight of your body sink toward the earth.

Step 3: Scan From Crown to Toes

Move your awareness slowly through your body.

- o Notice your forehead. Is it tight or relaxed?
- o Your jaw. Let it unclench.
- o Your shoulders. Let them drop.
- o Your chest. Is your breath shallow or full?
- o Your abdomen. Can it expand without tension?
- o Your legs and feet. Feel the ground holding you.

Don't judge what you find—observe. Each area of tension is simply a story asking to be heard.

Step 4: Listen for Wisdom

When you encounter tightness, ask:

"What are you trying to tell me?"

The body often answers softly: I'm tired. I'm afraid. I need rest. I need love.

Breathe compassion into that space.

Step 5: Close With Gratitude

Thank your body for carrying you through everything it has survived. Whisper, "You're safe now."

Repeat daily or before sleep. Over time, you'll begin to notice subtle shifts—ease replacing tension, peace replacing vigilance.

This is the nervous system learning that healing isn't a thought; it's a feeling.

Reflection Prompt: What Is My Body Saying?

After your body scan, journal the answers to these questions:

1. What sensations did I notice most strongly?
2. Where in my body do I carry stress, and when does it appear?
3. What message might that area hold?
4. What practices or environments help my body feel safe and open?
5. What would it look like to live today from that place of safety?

This process builds somatic literacy—learning the language your body speaks so you can respond with understanding rather than frustration.

The Physiology of Presence

Presence is physiology. When your nervous system is regulated, your prefrontal cortex (the rational, compassionate part of your brain) stays online. You respond instead of react. You listen instead of defending. You become a safe space in motion.

Embodiment, then, is not mystical—it's measurable. Heart-rate variability improves, digestion steadies, and inflammation lowers. Your biology mirrors your beliefs. You are literally shaping your health with your awareness.

Presence isn't passive; it is power made peaceful.

From Individual to Collective Embodiment

I've seen how embodiment changes rooms. In my own home, in community spaces, and especially in circles of shared healing, one regulated body shifts the tone for everyone else. When I slowed my breath, others followed. When I paused instead of reacting, conversations softened. I realized embodiment isn't private—it's relational. Your body teaches others what safety looks like without ever saying a word.

When one person lives embodied, they help others remember how. Families mirror each other's nervous systems; communities reflect the tone of their leaders.

If anxiety can spread, so can peace.

Imagine workplaces where leaders pause before reacting, homes where breath is the first response rather than blame, and communities that model stillness rather than speed.

This is how RISE becomes culture—when balance is not taught, but felt.

Embodied people don't preach peace; they carry it. They don't force trust; they represent it. This is how the RISE movement grows—not by programs, but by presence.

When the Body Finally Feels Safe

For a long time, I thought healing would feel dramatic—breakthroughs, clarity, resolution. Instead, it felt quieter. My body sighed more often. My sleep deepened. My reactions slowed. Safety didn't announce itself; it settled in. That's when I understood: healing isn't a moment. It's a nervous system learning it no longer has to prepare for harm.

Safety is the soil of transformation. Healing accelerates the moment the body stops expecting harm. In that safety, metabolism regulates, the immune system strengthens, and emotions integrate. This is why healing often begins with sighs, tears, and yawns—they're the nervous system's way of saying, "I can rest now."

When the body finally feels safe, the spirit feels heard. The heart expands. The mind quiets. And life begins to flow again.

Embodiment as Worship

Every culture has known this truth: movement and stillness are sacred languages. Bowing, dancing, kneeling, breathing—these are acts of reverence.

In Hebraic tradition, worship was whole-being participation: heart, mind, soul, and strength—the body itself.

Modern spirituality sometimes forgets that holiness is physical, too. To eat well, to breathe fully, to rest deeply—these are sacred acts.

When you walk gently on the earth, you are praying with your feet.

When you breathe consciously, you are aligning with the divine breath that first filled Adamah (the living earth/soil from which humanity was formed).

When you stand tall in truth, you are proclaiming belief without words.

Your body is the first temple you were given.

To honor it is to worship the One who made it.

Reflection Prompt

"Where does my body still carry a story my mind has outgrown?"

Sit with this question, not to analyze but to listen.

When that story rises—through tightness, ache, or tears—don't force it away. Let it speak. The moment you listen, it begins to loosen.

Embodiment isn't about perfection or performance.

It's about returning home to yourself, so you can walk in truth with others.

When the body remembers what the mind forgot, you become whole again—rooted, intentional, strong, and energized.

That is the beginning of balance.

Chapter 19 — Healing Together: The Power of Community

For much of my life, community felt complicated. I longed for connection, yet learned early that closeness could come with conditions. I learned how to be present without being fully seen, helpful without being held.

Even in adulthood, when relationships fractured—especially within my own family—I felt the ache of disconnection at a nervous-system level. Healing alone was possible to a point, but it was never complete. I could regulate myself, but I couldn't *relearn safety* without others.

What finally became clear was this: isolation didn't make me strong. It made me vigilant. Community, when it was safe and honest, is what allowed my body and spirit to exhale.

Healing was never meant to be a solo journey.

From our first breath, we are wired for connection. The newborn's heartbeat slows when held. The grieving person's tears ease when embraced. The isolated spirit begins to revive the moment another voice says, "Me too."

We are communal creatures in design and in destiny. The nervous system itself depends on relationships to regulate. Biology confirms what the soul already knows—belonging is medicine.

RISE began as one person's restoration story, but it became a movement the moment others gathered around the table and said, "I need this too." That gathering—whether in a living room, online, or around a Sabbath meal—is where theory turns to transformation.

Belonging: The Original Medicine

There were seasons when belonging felt theoretical—something I believed in more than experienced. After relational betrayal, I noticed how easily my nervous system interpreted closeness as risk.

I wanted connection, but my body stayed guarded. What slowly rebuilt trust wasn't perfection or agreement; it was consistency. Showing up week after week with people who didn't demand performance, didn't rush healing, and didn't weaponize vulnerability rewired something deep. Belonging didn't fix the pain, but it made it survivable. It reminded me I didn't have to carry everything alone.

Long before wellness programs, there were communities that healed simply by being together. Villages sang while they worked, neighbors shared harvests, and families ate from the same bowl. Connection wasn't an appointment—it was the atmosphere.

Modern life, however, has replaced belonging with busyness. Many of us have thousands of digital contacts but few embodied connections. Loneliness has become an epidemic, raising stress hormones, suppressing immunity, and shortening lifespan. The research is sobering: chronic social isolation increases mortality as much as smoking fifteen cigarettes a day.

Spiritually, disconnection is even costlier. We forget who we are when we're not mirrored by others who remember. We need someone to say, "You're still worthy," when shame says otherwise; someone to remind us of purpose when exhaustion whispers, "Give up."

Belonging doesn't erase struggle—it makes it survivable.

The Neuroscience of Connection

I didn't need neuroscience to tell me that safe presence heals—I felt it before I understood it. There were moments in shared spaces where my breath slowed simply because someone else was steady. No advice. No fixing. Just regulated presence. Over time, I realized my body was learning through experience what my mind already believed: that safety can be mutual. That not every connection demands defense. Biology gave language to what my body had already begun to trust.

When we experience safe relationships, the ventral vagal branch of the nervous system activates. Heart rate steadies, digestion improves, cortisol lowers, and oxytocin—the bonding hormone—rises. In short, we heal.

Psychologists call this co-regulation. It means our nervous systems literally synchronize with those around us. One calm presence can settle an entire room; one anxious person can unsettle it. This is why finding regulated, grounded people matters—healing spreads both ways.

Connection changes brain chemistry as powerfully as medication. In a healthy community:

- o The amygdala (fear center) quiets.
- o The prefrontal cortex (logic and empathy) re-engages.
- o The dopamine system (motivation and joy) re-awakens.

We feel safe enough to grow.

In trauma recovery, this is everything. Safety with another person re-teaches the body that the world can be trusted again.

How Belonging Sustains Change

I've learned that personal insight doesn't always survive pressure. There were times I knew what was healthy, what was true, what was aligned—yet without support, old patterns crept back in. Community didn't keep me accountable through correction; it kept me anchored through companionship. When others remembered my intentions on days I felt tired or discouraged, it gave my nervous system a place to land. Change didn't feel so fragile when it was shared.

Anyone can make temporary improvements through willpower. But only belonging creates stability. Change sustained in isolation often collapses under stress. Community provides accountability, encouragement, and perspective. It is the scaffolding that holds the transformation while it solidifies.

When you eat, pray, or think differently, it disrupts old patterns. Without support, the pull of the familiar can feel stronger than the call of freedom. But when others walk with you, momentum replaces fear.

Accountability isn't control; it's companionship with intention. It says, "I see your potential, and I'll hold space for it until you can."

That's the heartbeat of the RISE Circle.

RISE Circle: Healing in Rhythm

The RISE Circle began as a program. It was structured, intentional, and designed to support people in building healthy eating habits through shared learning. But something changed when the group was regathered. What had once been primarily instructional became relational. The framework stayed, but the atmosphere shifted. People didn't just show up to learn concepts; they came carrying real lives, real fatigue, real questions, real stressors.

As trust grew, the circle became less about delivery and more about presence. I found myself facilitating differently—not as someone dispensing answers, but as someone stewarding space. The program became a place where truth could be spoken safely, where balance was practiced together, and where healing moved from theory into lived experience.

The RISE Circle was born from the same soil as this book—real people seeking balance in the middle of real life. The RISE Circle embodies the four anchors: Rooted, Intentional, Strong, and Energized.

> **Rooted** — Every gathering begins with a check-in.
>
> Before diving into the week's topic, we take a few minutes to reconnect as humans. "How has your week been? What's on your mind today?" This simple pause helps everyone arrive fully, bringing their honest selves into the space without pressure or performance.

Intentional — Discussion flows from a chosen theme.

Nutrition, emotional healing, rest, sleep, movement, purpose—our conversations are guided by topics that support whole-being wellness. I regularly ask the group for input on what they want to explore, but most weeks I curate the theme myself, often drawing from what surfaced in our previous conversations. Everyone speaks from personal truth, not pretense.

Strong — Honest sharing requires courage.

I learned early on that vulnerability carries risk, especially when truth has been used against you. That's why I don't take courage lightly in these spaces. When I share first, it's not just to set an example—it's to lower the nervous system temperature in the room. I've watched people's shoulders drop when they realize they don't have to impress anyone. Strength in community isn't dominance or certainty; it's the willingness to be seen without armor.

Boundaries are honored; confidentiality creates safety. Strength here means vulnerability, not armor. As the facilitator, I often go first—sharing my own reflections from the week—because I've learned that when I lead with openness, it creates space for everyone else to breathe a little deeper and share more freely.

Energized — We end with lightness.

While we don't close with formal practices like prayer, breathwork, or meditation, our conversations often wind down with gentle laughter, shared encouragement, or a final reflection. The goal is simple: that everyone leaves a little lighter, more supported, and more energized than when they arrived.

These circles are not therapy sessions or church substitutes—they are ecosystems of encouragement. Within them, stories become seeds. One person's breakthrough waters the dry ground of others.

When practiced regularly, community rhythm becomes a biological regulator. People sleep better. Anxiety lessens. Even inflammation markers drop when individuals experience consistent emotional safety.

The Geometry of Connection: The Circle Itself

Why a circle?

Because circles have no hierarchy and no edges, every voice matters, every person faces the center, and energy flows continuously. In indigenous and Hebraic traditions, the circle symbolizes covenant—unbroken, eternal, inclusive.

The RISE Circle mirrors creation's own pattern: the orbit of planets, the rings of trees, the cycles of breath. It invites participation, not perfection.

When one member falters, the others carry the rhythm until they can re-enter. This is how balance becomes collective—each heart beating in time with the others, each life becoming a note in the symphony of wholeness.

Sacred Accountability

Accountability in RISE Circles isn't about measurement—it's about mindfulness. Members check in, not to judge progress, but to notice rhythm:

Are you resting as much as you're reaching?

Are you eating in alignment with your body's needs?

Are your thoughts kind, your pace humane?

These questions don't accuse; they awaken. They help participants return to awareness before imbalance becomes burnout.

In psychological terms, this creates feedback loops that sustain habits. In spiritual terms, it forms a pattern of wholeness—an invitation to practice life-giving habits in community.

The Physiology of Shared Joy

Joy is one of the most healing communal experiences. Laughter releases endorphins, increases oxygen flow, and strengthens immune function. Collective joy also dissolves shame—the emotion most likely to isolate.

When people celebrate each other's victories, dopamine reinforces motivation to continue. The body learns that healing feels good, not heavy. Joy becomes the nervous system's new normal.

Every RISE Circle meeting ends with a sense of what's growing. There's no formal gratitude round, but there is often a quiet awareness of progress—feeling a little lighter, gaining clarity, naming a breakthrough, or simply recognizing the strength it took to show up. These small moments of growth weave hope back into daily life.

When Community Hurts

I know firsthand that community can wound. When trust is broken—especially by those who share history or blood—the body remembers. That's why a safe community must be intentional, not assumed. Healing spaces don't demand participation; they invite it. They honor pacing, consent, and boundaries. I've learned that not every group deserves your story, but the right one will treat it as sacred. Safety is not automatic—it's cultivated.

For many, the idea of community brings ambivalence or fear. Past experiences with judgment, gossip, or betrayal leave scars. The nervous system remembers those, too.

A healing community must therefore be trauma-informed. It recognizes that people come carrying invisible stories. Safety, consent, and compassion are non-negotiable. The goal is never to fix others, only to witness them with respect.

In a safe community:

- o Sharing is an invitation, not an obligation.
- o Advice is replaced with empathy and shared experiences.
- o Prayer can be offered, but not imposed.
- o Silence is honored as much as speech.

When practiced this way, belonging itself becomes the antidote to the loneliness that once wounded us.

The Spiritual Dimension of Togetherness

In the Hebraic worldview, community (kehillah) is not optional—it's necessary, and it's sacred. GOD's presence dwells in the midst of gathered hearts, not isolated efforts. The early believers met in homes, shared meals, confessed weaknesses, and celebrated feasts—all rhythms of shared life.

When people align with divine design, even community follows natural law: giving and receiving, speaking and listening, work and rest. Each person reflects the Creator's image in a unique way, and together they reveal facets no one person could alone.

RISE Circles continue that tradition in modern form. They are reminders that wholeness multiplies in fellowship. You cannot practice peace in theory; you must practice it with people.

Practical Ways to Build Healing Community

1. Start Small. Two or three people meeting regularly can shift entire emotional ecosystems. Focus on consistency over size.
2. Set Intention. Begin each meeting with one word or verse that grounds the group's focus.
3. Share the Space. Everyone gets equal time; listening is as sacred as speaking.
4. Hold Confidentiality. Safety allows vulnerability. What's shared stays within the circle.
5. End with Renewal. Breathwork, gratitude, or a brief reflection closes the nervous system loop in peace. Our Circle usually ends in gratitude.
6. Check Energy, Not Perfection. Instead of "Did you meet your goal?" ask, "How does your energy feel this week?"
7. Celebrate Progress. Joy fuels continuation.

In time, these practices cultivate what psychologists call secure attachment—the inner knowing that you are safe and seen even when imperfect.

The Science of Mirroring

Human brains contain mirror neurons—cells that fire both when we act and when we observe someone else acting. Watching another person live calmly or courageously literally trains our own brain to do the same.

That's why community accelerates transformation: embodiment is contagious.

When someone demonstrates healthy boundaries, forgiveness, or self-care, others internalize that model. Seeing balance creates the belief that balance is possible.

Every RISE Circle becomes a mirror of collective potential—the place where balance is not just taught, but caught.

From Circles to Culture

I've seen how embodied healing doesn't stay contained. What shifts in one person begins to echo outward—into homes, parenting, partnerships, and workspaces. When I changed how I rested, spoke, and set boundaries, my household felt it. When RISE participants carried that regulation back into their families, it multiplied. Culture doesn't change through slogans; it changes through nervous systems that no longer live in survival mode.

As individuals heal, the culture shifts. Homes change tone; children absorb new emotional languages; workplaces grow more humane.

This is the larger vision of RISE—that wholeness becomes the norm, not the exception.

Imagine if our calendars honored rest as much as hustle, if community gatherings prioritized restoration over entertainment, if wellness wasn't a luxury but a lifestyle rooted in love.

Movements that endure begin with ordinary people living with extraordinary consistency. One balanced life at a time becomes a balanced community, then a balanced culture.

When You Forget Who You Are

There are still days when I forget. Days when old patterns whisper loudly, when fatigue dulls clarity, when isolation tempts me to retreat. That's when community matters most. Not to fix me—but to remind me. Healing doesn't require constant strength; it requires a connection that endures weakness. Community is where memory is shared, and truth is held until you can hold it again yourself.

There will still be days of fatigue and doubt. Healing is cyclical, not linear. That's why community exists: to remind you when you forget.

> When your faith wavers, someone else's can hold the line.
>
> When your energy fades, their presence lends stability.
>
> When shame whispers lies, love speaks louder through familiar voices.

Balance doesn't mean never falling; it means knowing who will catch you.

Community is the net that grace weaves beneath every RISE journey.

Reflection Prompt

"Who holds me steady when I forget who I am?"

List the names—or even the roles—of people who anchor you. Then ask yourself how you might reciprocate. Wholeness deepens when care flows in both directions.

If the list feels short, don't despair. Begin with one genuine connection. Sometimes healing starts with a single honest conversation that says, "I'm tired of pretending."

Write one step you can take this week to strengthen or seek a connection:

Send a note of gratitude.

Invite a friend for a walk.

Join or start a RISE Circle.

Belonging begins with initiative born of hope.

Chapter 20 — The Energy of Alignment

For a long time, I chased energy without realizing I was leaking it. I mistook intensity for vitality and endurance for alignment. There were seasons when I could function well enough, yet felt strangely hollow—tired even on days when nothing was technically "wrong."

What eventually became clear was that my exhaustion wasn't from doing too much; it was from living out of sync with what I knew to be true. Alignment didn't arrive as a breakthrough moment. It arrived as quiet relief—the first time my outer choices finally stopped arguing with my inner knowing.

There is a quiet kind of power that comes when your inner world and outer world move in unison.

No forcing. No fragmentation. Just the hum of harmony that tells every cell, I am where I'm meant to be.

That is the energy of alignment—vitality, peace, and purpose flowing freely through a life lived in rhythm with truth.

It isn't mystical or elitist; it's the birthright of every human being. Alignment is not about control—it's about coherence. It's what happens when thought, belief, body, and action all agree.

When you are aligned, you don't have to generate energy; it arises naturally.

Energy as Vitality, Connection, and Peace

Energy, in its simplest form, is life in motion. It animates every heartbeat, every thought, every moment of awareness. Science calls it bioelectricity; faith calls it Spirit; psychology calls it presence. Whatever language you prefer, it is the same current moving through you and all creation.

When you are aligned, that current flows unhindered. When you are disconnected—through stress, resentment, self-judgment, or overexertion—it fragments. The result is fatigue, irritability, confusion, and loss of joy.

True energy, then, isn't measured in productivity, but in peace. You know you're aligned not when you're doing more, but when you're doing less and feeling fully alive while doing it.

This kind of energy doesn't burn out; it burns steadily.

It's not the caffeine rush that spikes and crashes; it's the quiet radiance of coherence between heart and habit, soul and schedule, purpose and practice.

The Spiritual Science of Alignment

I used to think alignment was a spiritual concept—something abstract and aspirational. But my body experienced it first. When I stopped forcing outcomes, slowed my breath, and let go of resistance, my nervous system responded immediately. Calm replaced vigilance. Focus returned. Alignment didn't feel mystical; it felt familiar, like remembering a rhythm I had always known but forgotten how to trust.

Neuroscience shows that coherence—when brain waves, heart rhythm, and breath synchronize—produces measurable calm and focus. This is known as heart-brain alignment. The heart sends more signals to the brain than the brain does to the heart, guiding emotional clarity and intuitive awareness.

In spiritual language, this is being "in tune."

Your body becomes an instrument through which peace is played.

The Hebrew word ruach means both breath and spirit. Breath is the biological carrier of energy; spirit is its meaning. Every inhale is a gift of vitality; every exhale, a surrender of control.

When you live in alignment, you stop resisting the flow of ruach through you. You become an open channel for divine rhythm to move as rest, work, love, or laughter—whatever the moment calls for.

Sacred Ordinary Moments

Some of the most profound shifts in my energy didn't happen during prayer or retreat, but in the middle of ordinary tasks. Washing dishes without rushing. Walking without headphones. Folding laundry with intention instead of resentment. When I stopped hurrying through life to get to the "meaningful" parts, energy stopped draining away. Presence restored what striving never could.

Most of life's energy losses happen not in crises but in the ordinary rush between moments—checking messages, worrying over small things, multitasking meals, or rushing through joy. But sacred energy is cultivated in the same ordinary spaces when attention returns to presence.

Alignment doesn't require monasteries or mountaintops; it grows in kitchens, gardens, and car rides. It's the way you pause before responding, the way you breathe before deciding, the way you notice beauty in the midst of routine.

Everyday acts can become energy rituals when they are infused with awareness:

- o Washing dishes becomes meditation when done with gratitude.
- o Walking to the mailbox becomes a prayer when you breathe in peace and exhale worry.
- o Folding laundry becomes alignment when you bless the hands that will wear each garment.

These small sacred pauses repair the fragmentation caused by constant motion. They restore what hustle drains.

The miracle isn't in the moment—it's in your attention to it.

Stillness as the Source

Stillness used to make me uncomfortable. Silence felt unproductive, and rest felt like something I had to justify. But as I practiced stillness—especially during seasons when life felt uncertain—I realized it wasn't emptiness I feared; it was listening. Stillness brought clarity without effort. It reminded me that I didn't have to push life forward for it to move. Sometimes alignment arrives only when you stop interfering.

Stillness is not the absence of energy; it's its renewal chamber. In stillness, you stop scattering yourself across a thousand distractions and return to your center. When you become still—whether through prayer, breathwork, or quiet reflection—the body switches from sympathetic arousal (fight-or-flight) to parasympathetic restoration (rest-and-repair). Energy is replenished, not spent.

Think of a lake: when the wind ceases, the surface stills, and reflection becomes clear. In the same way, your mind's stillness allows truth to reflect.

Stillness does not demand silence from the world; it invites silence within you. It is not withdrawal; it's return.

Every time you stop, breathe, and be, alignment is restored.

Creation as Connection

Nature became one of my most consistent teachers of alignment. Walking outside, gardening, standing barefoot on the ground—these moments recalibrated me faster than analysis ever did. Creation didn't demand explanations or productivity; it offered participation. Watching how effortlessly the natural world moved through cycles of work and rest helped me release my obsession with constant motion. Energy returned when I remembered I belonged to the same design.

Nothing restores energy faster than reconnecting with the natural world. The same force that moves through rivers, trees, and tides moves through you. When you touch the earth, breathe outdoor air, or feel sunlight on your skin, your cells literally recalibrate.

Grounding—walking barefoot on grass, soil, or sand—equalizes your body's electrical charge. Studies show it lowers inflammation, improves sleep, and stabilizes mood. Sunlight regulates the circadian rhythm and boosts serotonin levels. Time in nature lowers blood pressure and increases alpha brain waves associated with calm alertness.

But beyond the data, nature teaches energy balance by example.

The tree doesn't hurry; the river doesn't resist.

The flower opens when it's ready and rests when it's dark.

When you remember your belonging to creation, you stop striving for energy and start participating in it.

Joy as Frequency

Joy is not frivolous—it's fuel.

Joy didn't feel safe to me at first. After years of bracing for disappointment, ease felt suspicious. But as I practiced noticing small delights—laughter at the table, warmth of sunlight, moments of shared humor—my body responded with openness instead of collapse. Joy became evidence that alignment was working. It wasn't escapism; it was integration. My nervous system was learning that life no longer required constant vigilance.

When you laugh, sing, dance, or smile, your energy frequency rises. Cells communicate better; digestion improves; pain thresholds increase.

Joy recalibrates the nervous system faster than discipline ever could. It tells the body, "I am safe enough to celebrate."

Yet joy often feels unsafe for people who've spent years in survival mode. The nervous system, accustomed to vigilance, then mistakes joy for danger. That's why joy must be practiced—small doses at first, like reintroducing sunlight after darkness.

Take thirty seconds each day to notice one thing that delights you— a scent, a song, a texture, a memory. Let it linger. Let it fill your senses. That's energy alignment in action. Joy is not a distraction from healing; it's proof that healing is working.

When Energy Feels Blocked

When my energy stalled, it was rarely random. It usually pointed to something I wasn't acknowledging—resentment I hadn't named, grief I hadn't released, or a boundary I hadn't honored. Once I stopped judging these moments and started listening to them, energy moved again. Authenticity restored what pretending had drained.

Even in awareness, energy sometimes stagnates. Fatigue, irritability, or creative numbness are signals, not failures. They're your body whispering, "Something is misaligned."

Ask gentle questions:

> Am I holding onto resentment or guilt?
>
> Am I pushing past my natural limits?
>
> Have I neglected rest, movement, or nourishment?
>
> Do my actions align with my values?

Often, blocked energy stems from emotional congestion—unspoken truth, unreleased grief, unmet needs. When you express honestly (through tears, prayer, writing, or conversation), the blockage softens.

The nervous system thrives on authenticity. Pretending is the most significant drain.

When you live truthfully, energy returns without strain.

The Rhythm of Receiving

Learning to receive was one of the hardest lessons of alignment for me. I was comfortable giving, explaining, and accommodating—but receiving felt unfamiliar. When I allowed myself to accept help, kindness, and rest without deflection, energy deepened instead of dissipating. Receiving taught me that alignment isn't self-sufficiency; it's participation in a rhythm larger than myself.

Alignment isn't only about output; it's about openness. Many of us were taught to give endlessly but struggle to receive—with compliments, help, love, or rest. Yet receiving is half the rhythm of life.

> Inhale and exhale.
>
> Day and night.
>
> Work and rest.
>
> Giving and receiving.

Energy circulates only when both sides of the rhythm are honored. Refusing to receive breaks the current and creates an imbalance.

Practice saying "thank you" instead of "I'm fine." Let others' kindness restore you rather than deflect it. Allow yourself to be nurtured by beauty, community, and grace.

The moment you allow yourself to receive, alignment deepens.

The Energy of Alignment in Relationships

As my own alignment strengthened, my relationships changed—not because others changed, but because I did. I stopped over-explaining. Boundaries clarified themselves. Peace became my reference point. Even when others were dysregulated, I noticed that my grounded presence influenced the interaction. Alignment didn't control outcomes, but it stabilized the connection. I learned that harmony begins internally and radiates outward.

When your energy aligns with peace, it shifts how you connect with others.

- Communication becomes clear because defensiveness dissolves.
- Boundaries become natural because self-worth is secure.
- Love becomes generous because it's no longer a transaction; it's an overflow.

Alignment makes relationships spacious. You stop needing others to complete you and start sharing energy from fullness, not emptiness.

In family, friendship, or community, aligned energy creates harmony where once there was conflict. Even when others are unregulated, your grounded presence becomes an anchor.

This is the quiet influence of the aligned: they don't convince; they calibrate.

The Restoration Practice: Evening Gratitude Ritual

Every night, your body resets its energy systems. Hormones shift, cellular repair begins, and the mind processes the day's experiences. The evening gratitude ritual aligns you with this natural restoration process—uniting biology, belief, and peace before rest.

Step 1 — Dim and Disconnect

An hour before bed, lower the lights and silence digital noise. This signals the pineal gland to release melatonin. Let the world's volume fade so your inner rhythm can rise.

Step 2 — Breathe and Return

Sit quietly or lie in bed. Inhale through the nose for four counts, exhale through the mouth for six. As you exhale, imagine releasing all the static that accumulated from the day—words, worries, tasks. Whisper, "It is finished for now."

Step 3 — Gratitude Flow

Bring to mind three specific moments from the day that brought life. They don't need to be grand—perhaps sunlight on your skin, laughter with a friend, or a moment of clarity. Name them aloud or in writing.

As you recall each one, notice how your chest softens and warmth spreads. Gratitude shifts the body into parasympathetic recovery mode, lowering blood pressure and slowing heart rate.

Step 4 — Releasing the Heavy

Next, acknowledge anything that felt misaligned—conflict, exhaustion, missed intentions. Instead of replaying it, breathe compassion into it. Say, "This, too, can rest tonight."

Forgiveness, even of minor irritations, unclogs energy for renewal.

Step 5 — Bless and Surrender

Place a hand over your heart and whisper:

"May my energy return to peace.

May my body rest in alignment.

May I wake renewed in rhythm with life."

This ritual takes five minutes but resets your entire system. Sleep becomes deeper, dreams clearer, mornings calmer. It's the energy of alignment preparing you for another day of RISE living.

When Alignment Becomes Embodiment

There was a time when alignment required constant attention. Now it feels more like muscle memory. My body notices when something is off before my mind does. Peace alerts me when I'm aligned; tension alerts me when I'm not. I no longer chase energy—I steward it. Alignment has become less about correction and more about return.

The more often you return to this rhythm, the more automatic it becomes. Alignment no longer requires conscious correction; it becomes your default state.

> You begin to live more slowly but accomplish more.
>
> You move less but mean more.
>
> You rest deeper and wake clearer.
>
> You start to sense energy not as something you chase but something you steward.

Eventually, the line between spiritual and physical blurs completely. Breath feels like prayer. Movement feels like worship. Joy feels like a revelation. Ordinary life becomes sacred liturgy.

That is the energy of alignment: living as if every cell in your being remembers who you are and why you're here.

Reflection Prompt

"What small practice helps me feel most connected to peace, and how can I honor it daily?"

Journal this before bed tonight. It might be a walk at dusk, candlelight during prayer, music during meals, or quiet breath before sleep. Consistency is more potent than intensity.

Choose one ritual that restores your energy and make it your daily homecoming.

PART VI

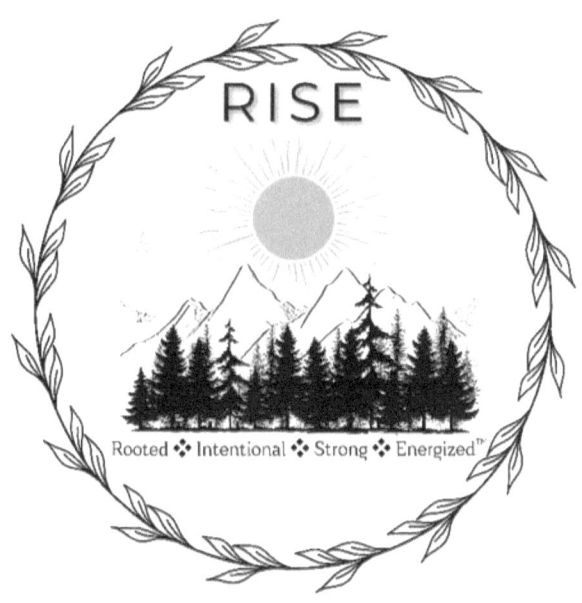

Integration and Invitation

Every path of healing eventually returns to simplicity.

After all the learning, practicing, and reflecting, there comes a quiet knowing: wholeness is not something you earn—it's something you remember.

The RISE journey has never been about perfection. It's about participation. It invites you to live awake—to move through each day aware of what is real, what is nourishing, and what is calling you back to balance.

Integration is where transformation takes root. It's when the four anchors—Rooted, Intentional, Strong, Energized—stop being ideas and start becoming instincts. It's when you no longer have to think your way into balance; you simply live it.

Perfection was never the point; rhythm was.

Because wholeness isn't a destination—it's a dance.

The final invitation of this book is to embody RISE not as a fixed framework but as a living circle. Let it evolve with your seasons. Let it breathe. Let it grow gentler. Let it meet you where you are, again and again.

Balance doesn't mean never wavering. It means returning—gracefully, honestly, and continually—to what is true.

You are already in the circle.

Now, you get to live it.

Chapter 21 — Dynamic Balance: Living the Circle of Wholeness

There were seasons when I thought balance meant finally getting everything under control. If I could just heal enough, rest enough, understand enough, life would stop wobbling. What I eventually learned—through grief, family rupture, and the ongoing practice of boundaries—was that balance isn't the absence of disruption. It's the ability to stay oriented when disruption comes.

The goal was never a perfectly even life; it was a responsive one. Dynamic balance didn't arrive when things settled down—it arrived when I learned how to return to center without abandoning myself.

When you first began reading, balance might have seemed like a faraway destination—a finish line at the end of exhaustion. But now you know: balance is dynamic, not static. It moves, breathes, and adjusts like the tides.

It isn't something to hold—it's something to flow with.

Dynamic balance means learning to live from your center even as life shifts around you. It's the art of staying flexible without losing focus, grounded without becoming rigid, peaceful without becoming passive.

This is the living philosophy of RISE.

Integrating the Four Anchors into One Practice

I didn't learn integration in theory; I learned it when one anchor collapsed and demanded support from the others. During seasons when emotional strain intensified—especially within family relationships—I couldn't rely on strength alone. I had to return to Rooted practices to stabilize my body and identity. When clarity wavered, I leaned into Intentional choices rather than forcing certainty. When exhaustion crept in, Energized didn't mean doing more—it meant restoring rhythm. Over time, I realized the anchors weren't separate skills to master; they were companions that carried one another when one grew tired.

The four anchors—Rooted, Intentional, Strong, Energized—are not four separate lessons but four expressions of one integrated life. They interact constantly, shaping one another in motion.

Think of them as the four seasons of wholeness, continuously cycling within you:

> Rooted: grounding in identity and belonging.
>
> Intentional: aligning thought and action.
>
> Strong: enduring through surrender.
>
> Energized: flowing with vitality and peace.

At any given time, one anchor may need more attention. Some days call for grounding; others, for courage; and still others, for rest. Living the RISE circle means honoring these natural fluctuations without judgment.

Integration happens when you stop compartmentalizing your healing. The same breath that centers you during meditation can also guide you in a meeting. The same awareness that brings peace at home can steady you in crisis. The same body that stretches in stillness can also express joy in motion.

Wholeness is not one part of you healed—it's every part of you cooperating.

Understanding Balance as Flow, Not Stasis

I used to interpret losing balance as failure. Any regression felt like proof I hadn't healed enough. But life kept proving otherwise. Stress resurfaced. Grief revisited. Energy dipped without warning. What changed wasn't the absence of wobble—it was my response to it. When I stopped panicking at the imbalances and started listening to them, balance became gentler. Each wobble pointed me back to what I needed next. The sway became information, not indictment.

In physics, balance is not the absence of movement—it's the harmony of forces. Even a tightrope walker sways. Their balance is alive because it responds.

Your balance works the same way. It's not about never falling out of rhythm; it's about noticing when you do and knowing how to return.

This is the essence of dynamic balance: *responsive alignment.*

You will lose rhythm sometimes. You will get tired, distracted, and discouraged. But imbalance isn't failure—it's feedback. Every wobble reminds you to come back to your center.

This realization releases perfectionism and replaces it with peace.

Because true balance isn't brittle; it's breathing.

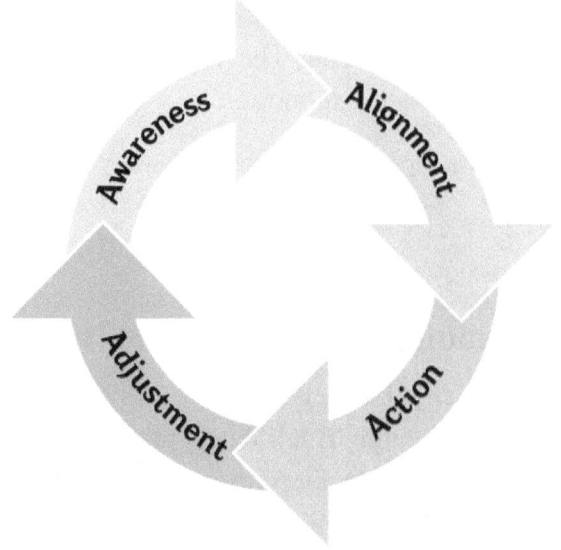

The RISE Feedback Loop:

Awareness → Alignment → Action → Adjustment

This loop didn't emerge for me as a clever tool; it formed organically through lived repetition. I noticed how awareness softened reaction, how small aligned actions restored peace faster than big declarations ever had. Sometimes the adjustment was as simple as stepping away from a conversation, going outside for breath, or choosing rest instead of explanation. Over time, this cycle became instinctive. Balance stopped being something I chased and became something I recalibrated—again and again.

Integration thrives on awareness. Once you know what throws you off-center, you can quickly begin recalibrating.

The RISE feedback loop is a simple process you can use daily or weekly:

1. Awareness – Notice where imbalance is showing up (in body, mind, emotion, or energy).
2. Alignment – Reconnect with truth. Ask, "What's most important right now?"
3. Action – Choose one small step that honors your values and rhythm.
4. Adjustment – Observe how it feels. If peace increases, continue. If strain increases, pivot gently.

Repeat as often as needed. This cycle transforms balance from theory into lifestyle.

Your RISE Rhythm in Real Life

These rhythms didn't unfold in ideal conditions. They unfolded in ordinary days—during mornings that began heavy, afternoons that tested patience, and evenings that needed closure. There were days when I didn't feel energized, yet honoring the rhythm still restored me.

Rooted mornings steadied me when the day ahead felt uncertain. Intentional pauses prevented burnout when emotions ran high. Strong afternoons reminded me I didn't need to push to prove resilience. Energized evenings became less about stimulation and more about letting go. The rhythm worked not because life was calm, but because it was honest.

Integration doesn't happen in isolation—it shows up in your daily flow:

Morning: Rooted in stillness. Begin with breath, gratitude, and grounding.

Midday: Intentional in motion. Move, nourish, refocus.

Afternoon: Strong in perseverance. Pace yourself with grace.

Evening: Energized in restoration. Release, reflect, and renew.

Each day becomes a miniature version of the greater circle. Each week, you revisit rest. Each season, you evolve. Each year, you rise again.

Living RISE in Relationships

Relationships were where dynamic balance was most tested. Alignment didn't mean avoiding conflict—it meant responding from clarity instead of compulsion. When I stopped trying to manage others' emotions and focused on regulating my own, boundaries became clearer, and communication softened.

Balance didn't guarantee harmony, but it preserved integrity. I learned that peace in relationships doesn't come from control or compliance; it comes from showing up whole and letting others respond from where they are.

When you live from dynamic balance, relationships shift, too. You stop expecting others to provide what you can generate internally. Peace replaces control, and compassion replaces comparison.

Rooted people create emotional safety.

Intentional people communicate clearly.

Strong people set healthy boundaries.

Energized people uplift others naturally.

Together, these qualities make relationships fertile soil for mutual growth instead of power struggles.

As more individuals live this way, family systems heal, communities flourish, and cultural patterns transform. This is how personal balance becomes collective wellness.

The Science of Integration: Coherence Across Systems

Integration is not just philosophical—it's physiological.

When you align your thoughts, emotions, and actions, your body becomes more efficient. Heart rate variability improves, inflammation lowers, and neural coherence increases. The brain, heart, and gut begin communicating fluidly. Decision-making becomes intuitive. Creativity rises.

This is what the HeartMath Institute calls "psychophysiological coherence." Spiritually, it's living in shalom—wholeness across all systems.

Dynamic balance means your internal orchestra is in tune. You no longer waste energy on inner conflict. Every system—biological, emotional, spiritual—plays the same song.

The Practice of Gentle Return

Gentle return became one of the most compassionate lessons of my life. There were moments when I recognized I had drifted— overgiving, overexplaining, overriding my body's cues. Instead of spiraling into self-criticism, I practiced returning. Sometimes that meant rest. Sometimes it meant truth. Sometimes it meant distance. Each return taught my nervous system that alignment was always available, even after missteps. That assurance changed everything.

No matter how aligned you become, life will keep inviting you back into chaos. Stress, grief, illness, or surprise will throw you off rhythm. That's not regression—it's the nature of complicated interactions as they occur in genuine relationships with real people.

The goal isn't to stay centered forever; it's to return more gracefully each time.

Think of it like waves meeting shore: they advance, retreat, and repeat—yet the shoreline remains. So too does your center.

When you falter, whisper, "I know my way back."

That confidence is the mark of integration.

Gentle return is both science (neuroplasticity) and spirituality (grace). The nervous system learns safety through repetition. The soul learns peace through forgiveness. Both together make balance sustainable.

The Circle of Wholeness

The circle stopped feeling symbolic when I realized I was already living it. I wasn't starting over when I returned to Rooted; I was continuing. Each pass through the circle carried more discernment. What once took weeks to notice now took moments. The circle didn't erase difficulty, but it did give it context. Life stopped feeling like a series of resets and started feeling like an expanding spiral.

The RISE Circle mentioned in earlier chapters now comes alive as a lifelong compass.

At the center is Presence—your still point of peace. Around it flow the four anchors, continuously orbiting:

Rooted → Intentional → Strong → Energized → Rooted again.

Each cycle deepens understanding. Each pass through the circle refines awareness.

When you feel scattered, you return to Rooted.

When you feel uncertain, you move to Intentional.

When life tests you, you embody Strength.

When the season lightens, you flow into Energized.

The circle ensures that you never have to start over—you simply continue.

Balance is not found in arriving but in revolving.

Self-Assessment Exercise:

"My Current RISE Landscape"

This exercise helps you visualize where you are in the circle right now.

Before you draw anything, begin with awareness. Pause, breathe, and reflect honestly on each anchor. Take your time. Your number is not a score—it is simply a signal. For each quadrant, reflect honestly.

Step 1: Reflect and Rate

Anchor	Questions to Reflect On	My Current Level (1–10)
Rooted	Do I feel grounded and connected to my identity, faith, and body?	

Intentional	Are my daily actions aligned with my deeper values and priorities?	
Strong	Am I resilient yet compassionate with myself during a challenge?	
Energized	Do I feel vibrant, rested, and in flow with my natural rhythms?	

Step 2 — Draw Your RISE Circle

Now that you have your four numbers, draw a circle and divide it into four quadrants labeled:

Rooted • Intentional • Strong • Energized

On each quadrant, mark your number outward from the center (1 close to the middle, 10 at the outer edge).

Then connect the points around the circle.

Your shape may be smooth or uneven, expansive or pulled inward in certain areas.

That shape reveals the truth of where you are currently in the circle; which areas are stable and which need work to bring you back to balance.

Step 3 — Notice What Your Circle Reveals

This visual snapshot shows your current RISE landscape. There is no right way for it to look.

There is only awareness, and awareness is where renewal begins.

Look at your circle when finished.

> Is it symmetrical or uneven?

> Where are you thriving?

> Where is care needed?

> Which anchors feel strong and steady?

> Which ones are calling for attention, tenderness, or renewal?

This visual snapshot shows your current RISE landscape. There is no score or success—only awareness. With awareness, renewal rises.

Then ask:

"Which anchor will I nurture this week to bring my circle back into rhythm?"

Small shifts—like earlier sleep, more precise boundaries, or intentional pauses—create powerful rebalancing.

Repeat the assessment monthly to see how your rhythm evolves. Your circle will never look perfect—and that's the beauty of living in balance dynamically.

Living Whole in an Unbalanced World

Living whole in an unbalanced world stopped feeling naïve once I experienced its stabilizing effect. My peace didn't depend on circumstances improving; it depended on alignment staying intact. The more consistently I returned to center, the less reactive I became to chaos around me. Balance became influence, not insulation.

You cannot control the chaos of the world, but you can choose the calm within it.

Dynamic balance means becoming a stabilizing presence in times of instability.

> Your peace becomes activism.

> Your alignment becomes influence.

RISE isn't about escaping the world; it's about engaging in it from a place of wholeness.

When you live rooted and intentional, strong and energized, you become a living demonstration that peace is possible here—now— in this world, not just the next.

From Framework to Flow

Integration didn't make life perfect. It made it navigable. I stopped demanding steadiness from circumstances and started cultivating it internally. The RISE framework didn't disappear—it became embodied. I no longer needed to remember what to do; my body and choices began remembering for me.

Every philosophy eventually dissolves into life. The RISE framework is never meant to confine you; it is intended to guide you back to yourself until you can move without it.

You don't have to follow every practice perfectly. You have to keep listening—to your body, your breath, your Creator, and the quiet call of balance.

Some days you'll dance through the rhythm; others you'll crawl. Both are sacred. What matters is that you keep returning.

That is integration.

That is wholeness.

That is the beginning—and the continuing—of balance.

Reflection Prompt

"How can I honor the rhythm of who I am becoming, rather than striving to perfect who I was?"

Write this at the top of your journal tonight. Let your response flow freely. Don't edit or analyze. Just listen.

Balance is not found by holding still—it's discovered in motion, shaped by grace.

The circle never ends, and neither does the invitation to rise again.

Chapter 22 — Wholeness Over Perfection

There came a moment in my healing journey when striving finally collapsed under its own weight.

I didn't decide to stop chasing perfection because I became enlightened or disciplined enough. I stopped because I was exhausted. All the self-help frameworks, the carefully managed routines, the constant effort to "do healing right" eventually revealed what they really were: elaborate ways to earn what I already feared I might not deserve.

Peace. Safety. Worth.

That collapse became the doorway.

What I discovered on the other side wasn't failure — it was relief. I wasn't broken. I never had been. I was becoming whole.

Perfectionism had promised arrival. Wholeness invited unfolding. And this, I realized, is where the RISE journey ultimately leads —

not to flawless execution, but to embodied peace. The kind that doesn't depend on productivity or proof, but presence.

The Shift from Self-Improvement to Self-Integration

For years, I approached wellness as self-improvement. My body was a project. My emotions were problems to manage. My faith became another metric to get right.

If I just healed enough, rested enough, understood enough — then I would be whole.

But healing didn't arrive through fixing. It arrived through integration.

Self-integration wasn't about adding better habits; it was about welcoming the parts of myself I had kept in exile. The strong part that survived. The soft part that still grieved. The disciplined part that built structure. The tired part that needed rest without justification.

I had spent years dividing myself into acceptable and unacceptable versions — the "strong one" versus the "emotional one," the "faithful one" versus the doubting one. Integration ended that war.

Wholeness came when I stopped asking which part of me was right and started listening to what each part needed.

Integration said something I had never heard before:

"You belong, even in your becoming."

The Illusion of Perfection

Perfection seduced me because it promised safety.

If I ate right, believed right, responded right, healed fast enough — maybe pain wouldn't find me again. Maybe loss wouldn't repeat. Maybe I could out run grief, shame, and unpredictability.

But perfection was never peace. It was performance dressed up as control.

I lived in constant vigilance — always assessing, correcting, optimizing. I couldn't rest because I was never "finished." I couldn't celebrate progress because there was always another benchmark. I couldn't fully connect because I was managing how I appeared.

Perfectionism fractured presence.

And slowly, quietly, my nervous system paid the price.

Scripture eventually reframed this for me. When Genesis calls creation tov — "good" — it doesn't mean flawless. It means functioning in harmony with purpose. Creation wasn't uniform; it was relational. Night and day. Work and rest. Joy and sorrow.

Wholeness was always the design.

I wasn't meant to be perfect — I was meant to be integrated. To live in right relationship with my body, my story, my Creator, and the rhythm of life.

When Perfection Becomes a Prison

Like many of us, I learned early that approval followed performance. That message didn't disappear in adulthood — it evolved. It sounded more spiritual. More responsible. More reasonable.

"If I just do better, I'll be enough."

That belief kept me in motion for years — overworking, over-explaining, over-giving. Underneath it all was fear: fear of rejection, fear of being misunderstood, fear of being seen as too needy, too much, or not enough.

My body carried that fear faithfully. Tight shoulders. Shallow breath. A nervous system that rarely stood down.

The tragedy was this: the harder I chased perfection, the more disconnected I became from myself.

Wholeness didn't begin when I achieved anything. It began when I stopped running. When I allowed imperfection to exist without immediate correction, my body exhaled. *Finally.*

That exhale was healing in real time.

Wholeness as Integration, Not Idealization

Wholeness didn't erase struggle from my life — it changed how I related to it.

Wholeness isn't about feeling good all the time. It is about no longer fighting myself when I didn't.

Wholeness is not a state of moral purity or flawless wellness; it's a way of being in relationship with truth. It's the realization that your story includes both the scar and the song—and that both matter.

When you integrate instead of "improving," you stop dividing life into "good days" and "bad days." Every day becomes a teacher and a companion.

I stopped labeling days as "good" or "bad." Every day became information. A teacher. A signal. Instead of asking What's wrong with me? I learned to ask different questions.

Instead of "How do I fix this?"

> I ask, "What is this showing me?"

Instead of "Why am I still struggling?"

> I ask, "What needs tending here?"

Instead of "When will I be healed?"

> I ask, "How can I honor the healing that is already happening?"

Wholeness doesn't require that everything feels easy; it simply means you stop fighting yourself in the process.

Embracing Imperfection as Proof of Humanity

Imperfection is not evidence of failure—it's evidence of life.

When you see yourself with that same compassion, your imperfections stop being obstacles and start becoming openings—cracks through which light enters.

I came to love the image of *kintsugi* — broken pottery repaired with gold. The cracks don't disappear; they become part of the design.

So did mine.

The fractures in my story — grief, loss, family rupture, seasons of exhaustion — weren't evidence of failure. They were golden threads in the mosaic of my becoming.

Scripture reinforced this truth again and again. Abraham doubted. Moses resisted. David failed publicly. None were remembered for flawlessness — only for the relationship.

The goal was never perfection.

It was always about connection.

The Science of Self-Compassion

Psychologist Kristin Neff defines self-compassion as treating yourself with the same kindness you would offer a good friend (https://self-compassion.org/).

Research consistently shows that self-compassion increases resilience, decreases anxiety, and even improves immune function. It lowers cortisol and raises oxytocin—the body's bonding hormone.

Self-compassion doesn't make you lazy; it makes you sustainable.

When you practice grace, you conserve the energy you would otherwise spend on self-criticism. That energy becomes available for creativity, purpose, and love.

Self-compassion is the nervous system's permission slip to rest. It says, "You're safe, even when imperfect."

Grace Over Grind

In a culture that glorifies the grind, choosing grace is a radical act.

Grace interrupts the hustle. It slows the pace and reorders priorities. It says:

"You don't have to prove your worth—you already are worthy."

Living from grace doesn't mean avoiding discipline; it means practicing discipline rooted in love, not fear.

The grind says, "Push harder."

Grace says, "Pause and listen."

The grind says, "Don't stop until you've earned it."

Grace says, "Rest—you're already enough."

Grace turns the wheel of performance into a circle of presence. It replaces exhaustion with flow. It transforms productivity into purpose.

Choosing grace over grind felt rebellious at first.

Grace slowed me down when hustle demanded speed. It reordered priorities I had mistaken for virtue. It reminded me I didn't need to prove my worth — I only needed to protect my peace.

Grace didn't eliminate discipline; it transformed it. Discipline rooted in love, not fear. When grace led, my body softened. My mind cleared. My spirit expanded.

That was alignment — grace embodied.

The Practice of Self-Integration

Integration is less about adding new habits and more about weaving existing wisdom into everyday life.

Here's a simple practice to help you move from fragmentation toward wholeness:

1. Notice Contradictions

Write down two qualities you've struggled to reconcile (e.g., "strong yet sensitive," "ambitious yet peaceful").

2. Name the Need

Ask each side what it's trying to protect or provide. Usually, both serve love in different ways.

3. Honor Both

Imagine them shaking hands. Affirm that both belong in your story.

4. Integrate in Action

Find one small way to live both today—perhaps by standing firm in truth while remaining gentle in tone.

The goal isn't to eliminate paradox but to embody it with peace.

Wholeness means you can hold opposites without splitting into sides.

The Spiritual Lens of Wholeness

In Hebraic understanding, shalom means far more than "peace." It signifies wholeness, harmony, and the absence of anything missing. Shalom describes the state in which all things function together as intended.

Wholeness, then, is sacred—it mirrors the Creator's design. When you return to inner harmony, you participate in cosmic restoration. Your body, mind, and spirit become microcosms of Eden restored.

The pursuit of perfection separated us from that harmony; the return to wholeness reconnects us.

Perfection says, "I must become divine."

Wholeness says, "The Divine is already within me."

That shift from striving to surrender is not slight—it's revolutionary.

The Wholeness Mindset in Practice

Here's how wholeness reframes daily life:

Old Paradigm	Wholeness Paradigm
Fix what's wrong	Integrate what's true
Hustle for worth	Rest in intrinsic value
Compete with others	Connect with others
Control outcomes	Co-create with grace
Hide flaws	Heal through honesty
Demand results	Honor the process
Fear failure	Learn through feedback

Living with this mindset transforms your energy, relationships, and resilience.

You stop reacting and start responding.

You stop comparing and start connecting.

You stop chasing and start creating.

This is how you live RISE beyond this book—it becomes reflex, not reminder.

Restoring the Rhythm of Enough

The most countercultural truth I learned was this:

Enough is sacred.

Enough sleep. Enough effort. Enough healing for today.

Not finished. Not perfected. Enough.

Honoring "enough" regulated my nervous system in ways no productivity system ever had. It taught me when to move and when to rest. When to engage and when to release.

Enough wasn't complacency — it was wisdom.

And when I honored it, my body responded with energy, my mind with clarity, and my spirit with joy.

Reflection Prompt

"Where can I choose grace over grind?"

Write freely. There are no "right" answers, no edits. Just notice where you feel pressure to prove and where peace is inviting you to pause.

Ask yourself:

> What would it look like to lead with love instead of fear?
>
> Where can I slow down without losing purpose?
>
> What am I trying to earn that is already mine?

Let your answers reveal where perfection still drives you—and where grace is asking to take the wheel.

Chapter 23 — When the Body's Clock and the Soul's Rhythm Agree

The Two Clocks I Learned to Listen To

For a long time, I thought exhaustion meant I wasn't trying hard enough. If I woke up tired, I pushed. If my mind raced at night, I blamed discipline. I didn't yet understand that my body and my soul were keeping two different kinds of time — and they were no longer speaking to each other.

The human body is always keeping time, even when we aren't aware of it. At the center of that quiet orchestration is a tiny cluster of neurons no bigger than a grain of rice: the suprachiasmatic nucleus, or SCN. Nestled deep within the hypothalamus, it acts like a conductor, raising and lowering its baton to the rhythm of light and darkness. Morning light tells the body, Rise. Begin again. Evening darkness softens the tempo: Slow down. Prepare for rest. *(For a deeper look at the SCN and circadian timing, see Appendix A.)*

The SCN listens to light as if it were language.

But the soul listens to something else entirely.

When Light Guides the Body but Meaning Guides the Soul

If photons guide the body's clock, the soul's rhythm is guided by meaning — by alignment, truth, purpose, safety, connection, and emotional honesty. I've woken many mornings when the sun said go, but my soul still lived in midnight. And I've lain in bed at night, biologically exhausted, while my soul refused to rest because something unresolved was still asking for attention.

The soul rises not because cortisol has increased, but because something inside feels awake. It rests not because melatonin surged, but because a sense of belonging has finally settled.

Modern life rarely allows these two clocks to synchronize on their own. I learned this the hard way.

There were seasons when my body was technically functioning — eating, moving, sleeping — while my soul carried grief, pressure, and unspoken truth. On the outside, nothing looked "wrong." Inside, everything felt off.

How Misalignment Shows Up Before It Shouts

Before an imbalance becomes a crisis, it whispers.

I've felt it as:

- o Foggy mornings after late nights under artificial light.
- o Anxiety that spikes at noon for reasons I can't immediately name.

- A heaviness at dusk after racing through a day with no pleasure or meaning.
- A deep exhaustion not from what I did, but from who I had to be to get through it.

These moments taught me something important: fatigue is often communication.

The body speaks through the SCN.

The soul speaks through emotion.

And when both are ignored, life becomes unsustainable.

What Science Can Measure — and What It Can't

Circadian science explains the biological side with remarkable clarity. When light enters the eyes at the wrong time — late-night screens, inconsistent sleep cycles, indoor living — the SCN becomes confused. Hormones are released out of order. Metabolism drifts. Mood destabilizes. Cognitive clarity dims. Immunity weakens. The body begins to feel like a poorly tuned instrument.

But soul rhythm follows a different kind of light. Its illumination comes from meaning.

When I lived out of alignment — saying yes when my body said no, carrying emotional wounds quietly, living according to expectations that weren't mine — my soul's inner clock began slipping. Time blurred. Energy dulled. Purpose faded. Joy felt distant, not because I was depressed, but because I was living out of season.

This kind of fatigue doesn't respond to sleep alone.

When the Two Clocks Disagree

I learned that a restless soul can override melatonin just as easily as a glowing screen. Emotional tension tightens the body. Unspoken truth raises cortisol. Unresolved grief interrupts rest.

When the body and soul fall out of sync, the consequences multiply:

> You're tired but wired.

> Exhausted yet unable to sleep.

> Functioning but not restored.

> Moving through days without inhabiting them.

I lived there longer than I want to admit.

What Alignment Actually Feels Like

But when the body's clock and the soul's rhythm agree, something quietly profound happens.

> Energy becomes effortless.

> Waking feels natural, not forced.

> Movement feels fluid, not pressured.

> Rest restores instead of interrupting.

> Emotions rise and settle with clean edges.

> Thoughts grow kinder.

> Decisions feel grounded rather than frantic.

This isn't productivity. It's coherence. It's the felt sense of being whole.

How I Began to Bring the Clocks Back Together

Alignment didn't arrive all at once. It came through small, honest shifts.

I began eating in ways that honored both nourishment and hunger. I moved my body in ways that felt joyful instead of punishing. I let emotions flow rather than compress them. I said yes to relationships that nurtured me and no to ones that drained me. I gave myself permission to rest without earning it.

Slowly, the SCN wasn't the only thing setting the pace. My soul began to steady the beat, too.

Biological Harmony Meets Existential Harmony

Scientists call circadian alignment biological harmony. I've come to think of soul alignment as existential harmony — the moment when who you are, what you believe, how you live, and what you desire begin pointing in the same direction.

When these harmonies meet, life gains an ease that doesn't depend on circumstances. Morning becomes more than routine. Light touches the eyes, and something inside awakens, too. Evening becomes more than a shutdown. The body slows, and the soul feels safe enough to follow.

This is why rest only works when it's honest.

The Gentle Questions That Restore Coherence

The invitation is never to perfection. It's awareness.

I've learned to ask:

Where are my clocks drifting apart?

Where is my body moving one way while my soul pulls another?

What am I forcing that needs alignment instead?

These questions don't accuse. They open.

Sometimes rhythm is lost for a day.

Sometimes for a season.

Sometimes for years.

Busyness, trauma, grief, comparison, chronic stress — all can disrupt the beat. But rhythm can be recovered. Gently. Compassionately. One aligned choice at a time.

When the body's time and the soul's truth begin to agree again, life doesn't become perfect. It becomes livable. And that agreement — quiet, embodied, and honest — is where healing finally holds.

Reflection Prompt

Where have you lost rhythm—with the day, the week, the season, or your years?
And what small shift would allow your body's clock and your soul's rhythm to agree again?

Chapter 24 — Begin Where You Are

Every ending in life is just another beginning disguised in softer light.

The RISE journey doesn't close here—it deepens. You've been walking toward something all along, but perhaps you've realized by now: there isn't a finish line waiting out ahead of you. It's home. This chapter is that homecoming—an invitation not to start over, but to start from within.

You're Not Starting Over — You're Coming Home

When people reach the end of a healing journey, they often whisper the same words: "I feel like I'm beginning again."

It's true, but not in the way they mean.

Beginning again doesn't mean returning to square one. It means returning to yourself—the version of you that existed before the noise, before the striving, before you were told you needed fixing.

You're not starting over; you're coming home. Coming home to your breath, your rhythm, your worth, your Creator's gentle design pulsing through your veins. Coming home to the truth that balance was never lost—it was simply waiting beneath the clutter of "shoulds" and "somedays."

Every practice, every reflection, every pause in this book has been a path back to presence. RISE was never about becoming something new; it was about remembering what you already are: Rooted. Intentional. Strong. Energized.

That's the secret no one tells you about transformation—it's more about returning than reinventing.

The Circle Brings You Back

In nature, everything circles back.

The sun rises and sets, tides ebb and flow, seasons bloom and rest.

So does the human heart.

When you complete a cycle of healing, it doesn't mean you've arrived—it means you're ready to rise into the next rhythm with greater wisdom and gentleness.

That's the pattern embedded in RISE itself: Rooted leads to Intention, Intention builds Strength, Strength awakens Energy, and Energy grounds you once again in Rootedness.

The circle never ends because growth never does. It's not an achievement—it's a relationship. Balance is not an object to hold; it's a friendship to nurture. Every day you live inside the circle, the circle lives deeper inside you.

A Gentle Call to Action

Many readers will finish this book with a mix of inspiration and hesitation.

They'll ask, "Where do I even begin?"

The answer is simple:

Right here. Right now.

Begin where you are—with the breath in your lungs and the ground beneath your feet. You don't need a perfect plan. You just need willingness.

Start with one micro-shift: a slower morning, a mindful meal, an evening of rest without guilt. Choose one anchor that feels inviting this week—Rooted, Intentional, Strong, or Energized—and let it lead you into rhythm again.

Transformation doesn't happen through grand gestures. It occurs in the gentle consistency of small choices made in awareness. Every sip of water, every deep breath, every act of honesty or gratitude is an act of beginning. You've already begun more times than you realize. The point isn't to rush forward—it's to move forward faithfully.

Living RISE Beyond the Page

The RISE philosophy was never meant to stay inside a book. It's meant to live in kitchens and gardens, in early mornings and late-night prayers, in workplaces and friendships, in laughter and quiet. It's meant to shape the way you move through the world—balanced, believing, embodied.

That's why The Beginning of Balance exists: to set a foundation for a new way of living, one that honors your humanity as profoundly as it honors your divinity.

RISE is more than a framework; it's a family of practices—a way of belonging to yourself, your Creator, and your community again. To live the RISE way is to remember that balance is both personal and collective. When one person lives in rhythm, the world around them begins to shift. You've felt it—those days when you walk in calm confidence, and others breathe easier just by being near you. That's what alignment does. It radiates. You are part of the quiet revolution of restoration—ordinary people learning extraordinary peace.

You Don't Have to Master It — Just Move with It

It's natural to feel a spark of motivation reading these pages—to want to fix everything all at once. But mastery is not the goal. Movement is.

RISE is a living philosophy precisely because it flexes with your humanity. Some seasons you'll feel deeply rooted; others you'll feel restless. Some days you'll rise strong; others you'll simply breathe. That's the beauty of rhythm—it makes space for both stillness and motion.

If all you can do today is breathe more mindfully than yesterday, that's balance in action. If all you can do this week is say no to one thing that drains you, that's alignment growing. If all you can do this month is keep showing up with honesty and grace, that's wholeness unfolding.

You don't have to climb a mountain.

You just have to keep walking—slowly, intentionally, faithfully.

Stay in Rhythm; Stay in RISE

When I first began this journey, I thought RISE was a wellness model. Now I see it for what it truly is: a mirror. It reflects the truth that balance isn't something you achieve—it's something you live in rhythm with.

Staying in balance means honoring the ebb as much as the flow. It means resting as fiercely as you rise. It means trusting that even when you lose your footing, the circle still holds you.

Staying in RISE means remembering that you are always part of something larger—an ongoing movement of restoration, grace, and embodied truth.

Whether you're journaling your reflections, gathering with your RISE Circle, or simply pausing to breathe between tasks, you are part of this living ecosystem of wholeness. This is not a theory anymore. This is you, alive in rhythm.

The Invitation

So, here we are—the end of one book and the beginning of the next.

The page will turn, but the path remains the same.

You have everything you need to begin again:

> A body that longs for restoration.

> A mind that is learning to rest in truth.

> A spirit that remembers its rhythm.

You are ready—not because you've mastered balance, but because you've met yourself in the process.

Now the question is not, "How far do I have to go?"

The question is, "How gently can I begin?"

Begin where you are—with what you have, with who you are, with the breath you're breathing now.

Closing Affirmation

I am rooted in grace,

intentional in growth,

strong in surrender,

and energized in peace.

I am not behind.

I am right on time.

I walk in rhythm with my Creator,

with creation,

and with my own becoming.

I don't need to start over.

I just need to begin again—

right here,

right now,

in RISE.

Stay in Rhythm. Stay in RISE.

When you close this book, take one slow breath.

Feel the air fill your lungs.

Feel your heartbeat align with your breath.

Feel the stillness beneath the movement.

That's balance.

That's home.

That's RISE.

And it begins—always—right where you are.

Epilogue — The Beginning of Balance

The end of one chapter in life is rarely an ending at all.

It is the quiet pause before a new rhythm begins to rise.

And if there is one truth this book has whispered from the first page to the last, it is this: balance isn't the goal. It's a way of being.

Wholeness doesn't wait at the finish line—it starts with the first breath of awareness, the smallest step toward presence, the simplest moment of choosing life again.

You've walked through portions of my story. In some way, it's also been yours—because every person who longs for peace, who tires of chasing perfection, who aches to feel whole again, eventually finds themselves here: standing in the space between exhaustion and awakening.

That space—right there—is sacred. It's the doorway of beginning.

The Moment Everything Changed

When I first began this journey, I was searching for answers. Answers for my health, for my mind, for my purpose. But answers alone don't heal. They only inform. Healing begins when knowledge becomes embodiment—when ideas take root in the soil of lived experience.

The moment that shifted everything for me wasn't a seminar or a diagnosis or even a revelation. It was a quiet moment of surrender. I had tried everything—every diet, every plan, every mindset—and I was still tired. I realized I was trying to become someone else's version of whole.

That's when I heard the whisper: "Begin where you are."

That phrase became the seed that grew into RISE.

The Birth of a Movement

RISE didn't begin as a brand or a book. It began as a conversation—a small circle of people talking honestly about their struggles with health, identity, and faith.

We weren't experts. We were explorers. Each of us had been burned out by systems—religious, medical, societal—that treated symptoms instead of souls. We needed something more human.

> Something that honored belief without demanding uniformity.

> Something that saw the body not as an obstacle to holiness, but as part of the sacred design itself.

From those conversations came four words that captured what we were trying to live:

Rooted. Intentional. Strong. Energized.

Those words became a framework, and that framework became a philosophy. Then the philosophy became a movement. Today, RISE is no longer just my story—it's ours.

The RISE Circles

I'll never forget the first RISE Circle meeting. It wasn't fancy—just a handful of us on Zoom, coffee mugs in hand, hearts cracked open from the week.

We talked about where we felt stuck, what small wins we'd seen, and what we were learning about rest, nourishment, or forgiveness. Some weeks, we cried. Some weeks, we laughed until our screens shook. And every week, something sacred happened: we remembered together.

RISE Circles are not support groups in the traditional sense. They are communities of remembering. Each person brings a story, a rhythm, a revelation. Together, we form harmony—a reminder that balance is not solitary, it's shared.

The circle teaches what life already knows: healing accelerates in the presence of belonging.

You don't have to rise alone.

Why Balance Must Begin in Community

We were never designed to self-regulate in isolation.

The nervous system finds safety through co-regulation—through eye contact, shared laughter, gentle tone, and compassionate presence.

When someone sits beside you and says, "Me too," your body exhales. Shame loses its grip. That's what happens in a community. That's what happens in RISE.

Balance begins within you, but it takes root in community. When others mirror your healing, your system learns to sustain it. That's why this movement matters because no one heals in a vacuum.

We rise together—or not at all.

The Sacred Middle

One of the hardest truths I've learned is that balance rarely feels like balance while you're living it. It often feels like the middle—messy, uncertain, constantly shifting. But that's where life actually happens: in the sacred middle between extremes.

> Between work and rest.

> Between ambition and surrender.

> Between confidence and humility.

The middle isn't mediocrity—it's mastery. It's where you learn to flow with what is, instead of fighting for what should be.

The sacred middle is the birthplace of grace.

That's why perfectionism doesn't belong in RISE—it has no room in the rhythm of becoming. You don't have to get it all right. You just have to stay in motion.

The Body as Messenger, Not Enemy

So many of us were taught to battle our bodies—to discipline them into submission or ignore them until they broke. But the body is not an obstacle to wholeness; it's a messenger of it. Every symptom is a signal, every craving a conversation, every ache a whisper.

When I began to listen to my body—not with fear, but with curiosity—I discovered that it wasn't sabotaging me. It was trying to lead me home.

Balance begins when you shift from blaming your body to befriending it. That's when energy returns, digestion improves, sleep deepens, emotions regulate, and clarity emerges—not because you forced it, but because you finally stopped fighting the very vessel through which healing flows.

Your body is not against you.

It's waiting for you to come back.

The Balance Between Faith and Science

One of the core distinctives of RISE is the bridge it builds between spirituality and psychology, between Scripture and science. You don't have to choose between faith and facts. Both reveal truth—just through different languages.

Science tells us how the body and mind function; faith reminds us why they matter. Science explains the nervous system; faith teaches peace beyond understanding. Science measures circadian rhythm; faith honors Sabbath rhythm. The two were never meant to be at odds. They're partners in the pursuit of wholeness.

This integration—of evidence and essence, research and revelation—is what makes RISE so powerful. It unites what religion and culture often divide. That unity is the very definition of shalom: everything in right relationship.

When Healing Becomes Overflow

There's a sacred turning point in every healing journey when you realize your transformation is no longer just about you.

> Your balance starts spilling over.

> Your peace becomes contagious.

> Your rest gives others permission to rest too.

Healing multiplies through presence. That's why RISE isn't content to stay within personal growth; it's meant to ripple into culture.

> Healthy people create healthy families.

> Healthy families create healthy communities.

> Healthy communities create a healed world.

That's the long vision of RISE—to become not just a wellness model but a cultural reformation, reminding the world that balance is the natural state of creation.

Living the Practice

If this book has been a conversation between your mind and your spirit, then what comes next is an invitation to embodiment—to make balance visible in motion.

> Practice it imperfectly.

> Practice it quietly.

> Practice it anyway.

Wake and stretch before your phone. Eat foods grown close to the earth. Rest when your body asks for it. Walk barefoot on soil and remember that you are dust and divine breath intertwined. Pause before speaking; breathe before reacting. Forgive faster. Laugh louder. Love slower.

Balance isn't hidden in rituals—it's found in responsiveness. It's not about doing more; it's about doing with awareness. Every small moment of mindfulness becomes an act of restoration.

The Next Evolution

What you've just completed is not a book you finished, but a record you began.

The Beginning of Balance Chronicles (a companion to this book) is a lived record and guided journal—one designed to help you notice your rhythms, name your patterns, and tell the truth about how balance is actually built through the RISE framework. Those pages were never meant to be mastered or completed. They exist to hold your experience as it unfolds.

From here, the journey can continue in different ways.

One path forward is the Seven-Year RISE Journey—a sequence of journals created to support steady, seasonal growth over time. This journey unfolds across years, not months, offering repeated opportunities to return to reflection, recalibration, and lived balance as life changes. Each season invites you to deepen how you live Rooted, Intentional, Strong, and Energized—not by striving, but by returning.

Alongside this journal journey exists a separate, but complementary resource:

The 9 Pillars of Whole-Being Wellness for a Balanced Life. This is not part of the journal sequence. It serves as a guidebook—offering structure, language, and practical clarity for those who want a deeper understanding of the principles that support everyday balance. Where the journals hold your lived experience, the pillars provide orientation when you want it.

These elements belong to the same ecosystem, but they are not the same thing. There is no required order, no pressure to engage with it all at once.

If these pages helped you lay the groundwork, the rest of the RISE ecosystem exists to support how you choose to continue living in balance.

There is no finish line here. Only an invitation to keep noticing, choosing, and returning—over time.

The Personal Becomes Collective

When RISE first began, I thought my story was unique. Now I see it's universal. We're all trying to reconcile the same tension: how to be spiritual and embodied, faithful and human, disciplined and gentle. We're all searching for the same middle path—the way back to balance. This movement is not about me. It's about we.

Every person who gathers in a circle, every journal entry written, every pause made with intention, becomes part of this living organism of wholeness.

RISE is not just a philosophy—it's a collective heartbeat.

And that heartbeat grows stronger with every person who chooses to listen.

A Personal Word of Gratitude

Before we turn the page into what's next, I want to say thank you—for reading these words, for trusting your journey, for opening your heart to possibility. You are the reason this movement exists. Your willingness to keep showing up—messy, real, hopeful—is the proof that healing is possible.

If this book has reminded you that your story matters, that your body is good, that your faith can be gentle and still strong—then every word has found its purpose. Because healing multiplies through honesty, and you've had the courage to walk through yours.

Thank you for walking with me.

The Beginning of Balance

The title of this book was never meant to be clever—it was meant to be prophetic. This really is the beginning of balance. Every moment you pause to breathe, every choice you make with awareness, every time you choose presence over perfection, you are participating in something holy.

This beginning is not small. It is revolutionary. Because a balanced person shifts everything and everyone around them. They walk into rooms and bring calm where chaos once ruled. They love without agenda. They work without burnout. They rest without guilt. And through them, the world remembers that healing is possible.

That's how light returns—one aligned heart at a time.

Final Blessing

May you rise with grace and rest without guilt.

May your roots grow deep in truth, and your branches stretch wide with compassion.

May you find rhythm in your breath, courage in your stillness, and freedom in your imperfection.

May you carry the calm of wholeness into every space you enter, and may others remember what peace feels like just by standing near you.

You are part of the restoration. You are the beginning of balance.

Stay in rhythm.

Stay in grace.

Stay in RISE.

A Closing Thought

The RISE journey never really ends. It widens. Each season, each breath, each step becomes another way to live in harmony with yourself, your Creator, and the world around you.

Afterword: Walking It Out

If you've reached this point in *RISE: The Beginning of Balance*, take a deep breath. You've just walked through years of lived lessons — not just mine, but pieces of your own reflected back through these pages.

This book began as a story of survival, but it became something much deeper: a story of remembering. Remembering what the body already knows, what the spirit already longs for, and what the heart has been whispering all along — that you were made for wholeness.

Balance isn't a finish line you cross. It's the way you move through your days — one steady inhale, one honest reflection, one small act of alignment at a time. You won't always feel steady, but steadiness grows in the returning. Every pause, every breath, every "try again" is proof that your rhythm is still alive.

The RISE framework — Rooted, Intentional, Strong, and Energized — was never meant to be a checklist. It's a way of being. A gentle compass that reminds you to look inward when the world feels loud, to anchor in truth when life pulls you off course, and to reconnect when you start to drift.

There will be days when you forget. Days when you rush, react, or lose your footing. Don't call that failure — call it feedback. Every moment of imbalance is your body and soul calling you home.

You have permission to grow slowly.

You have permission to rest when the world demands motion.

You have permission to be both a masterpiece and a work in progress.

As you step forward, I hope you will not only remember the words but also embody them. Let the ideas in these chapters translate into breath, movement, nourishment, and connection. Let them shape the choices that shape your life.

And when you find yourself in the company of others who are still searching — for peace, for purpose, for health, for meaning — share what you've learned here. Tell them about the rhythm that changed you. Tell them about the freedom found in alignment because the world doesn't need more perfection. It needs people who are present.

May this not be the end of your RISE journey, but the beginning of living it out — through the food you eat, the words you speak, the love you give, and the pauses you protect.

Keep listening to your inner wisdom.

Keep honoring your body's natural rhythm.

Keep rising, gently, with grace.

You don't have to do it all at once.

You just have to begin — right where you are.

With gratitude and hope,

Angel Tate Keaton

Founder, Healthy in Heart Media

Creator of RISE Whole-Being Wellness

Appendix A: Adding the Science of Rhythm: The Circadian Layer

1. Daily Renewal → The 24-Hour RISE Cycle

Core Idea: Every cell in the body runs on a near-24-hour clock orchestrated by the suprachiasmatic nucleus (SCN) in the brain's hypothalamus. Light, food, movement, and social connection act as *zeitgebers* ("time-givers") that keep it synchronized.

Mind-Body Areas Affected

System	What the Rhythm Regulates	How to Apply the RISE Principles
Brain & Mood	Cortisol and melatonin cycles shape alertness, focus, and emotional stability.	*Rooted:* wake with light exposure, *Intentional:* plan deep work mid-morning, *Strong:* pause mid-afternoon instead of pushing through, *Energized:* dim lights 2 h before sleep.
Metabolism & Digestion	Insulin sensitivity, gut motility, and enzyme activity peak earlier in the day.	Eat main meals in daylight; avoid late heavy meals; use a gentle fasting window for nightly repair.
Hormones & Immunity	Growth hormone, thyroid hormones, and immune cell release follow circadian waves.	Align movement and rest with these patterns—morning motion, evening recovery.
Detox & Repair	Nighttime lymphatic and liver cleansing depend on darkness and rest.	Keep nighttime screens off; honor true rest as a healing practice.

2. Weekly Renewal → The Rest-Repair Rhythm

Biologically, humans cycle through seven-day patterns in immune response, heart-rate variability, and even skin renewal (called *circaseptan* rhythms).

Practical tie-in: Your "Sabbath Rhythm of Healing" becomes the *weekly recalibration of the internal clock*—a literal metabolic reset through stillness, social connection, and reflection.

3. Seasonal Renewal → The Light-Length Cycle

As daylight length shifts, melatonin timing and serotonin levels change.

- Winter: More melatonin → greater need for rest, warmth, and internal focus.
- Spring/Summer: Longer days → higher dopamine and vitamin D → natural drive for creativity and movement.

Application: Seasonal renewal teaches you to adapt food, movement, and emotional focus to each season rather than resist it.

4. Lifelong Renewal → The Hormonal & Chrono-Aging Cycle

Over decades, circadian amplitude (the strength of those rhythms) weakens, which explains midlife fatigue, insomnia, and emotional flattening.

RISE integration: lifelong balance = preserving rhythm strength through light exposure, consistent meal timing, meaningful routine, and emotional flow.

Appendix B: Resources & Recommended Reading

A Curated Collection for Whole-Being Wellness

The following books, teachers, and organizations have influenced my own healing journey and the creation of the RISE Framework. They represent a meeting place of science, spirituality, psychology, and practice — an open table where truth, compassion, and curiosity meet.

The Science of Balance & Healing

Exploring how biology, rhythm, and environment shape wellness.

- **Dr. John McDougall** — *The Starch Solution*
- **Dr. Caldwell Esselstyn** — *Prevent and Reverse Heart Disease*
- **Dr. T. Colin Campbell** — *The China Study*
- **Dr. Neal Barnard** — *Your Body in Balance*; *The Power Foods for the Brain*
- **Dr. Doug Lisle & Dr. Alan Goldhammer** — *The Pleasure Trap*
- **Dr. John Bergman** — Educational videos on holistic anatomy and body systems
- **Dr. Michael Greger** — *How Not to Die*; *How Not to Age*
- **Dr. Andrew Huberman** — *Huberman Lab Podcast* (neuroscience and circadian rhythm)
- **Matthew Walker** — *Why We Sleep* (understanding the body's natural rhythms)

The Psychology of Transformation

Understanding thought patterns, trauma, and emotional healing.

- **Dr. Caroline Leaf** — *Switch On Your Brain*
- **Brené Brown** — *The Gifts of Imperfection*; *Atlas of the Heart*
- **Dr. Gabor Maté** — *The Myth of Normal*; *When the Body Says No*
- **Peter Levine** — *Waking the Tiger: Healing Trauma*
- **Deb Dana** — *Polyvagal Theory in Therapy*
- **Dr. Edith Eger** — *The Gift: 12 Lessons to Save Your Life*
- **James Clear** — *Atomic Habits* (small shifts that build sustainable change)
- **Jon Kabat-Zinn** — *Wherever You Go, There You Are* (mindfulness and presence)

Spiritual Restoration & Hebraic Understanding

Bridging faith, creation, and the sacred rhythms of life.

- **Ross K. Nichols** — *The Moses Scroll*; Horeb Institute
- **Rabbi Jonathan Sacks** — *To Heal a Fractured World*
- **Skip Moen** — *Spiritual Restoration* and daily Hebrew word studies
- **Tovia Singer** — *Let's Get Biblical* (contextual understanding of faith)
- **Richard Rohr** — *Falling Upward* (spiritual maturity and transformation)
- **Horeb Institute** — For those pursuing Hebraic truth and renewal

Emotional Wellness & Self-Compassion

Learning the gentle art of grace, boundaries, and restoration.

- **Kristin Neff** — *Self-Compassion: The Proven Power of Being Kind to Yourself*
- **Dr. Nicole LePera** — *How to Do the Work*
- **Dr. Dan Siegel** — *The Whole-Brain Child*; *Mindsight*
- **Glennon Doyle** — *Untamed* (living honestly in alignment)
- **Tara Brach** — *Radical Acceptance*; *True Refuge*
- **Sharon Salzberg** — *Lovingkindness: The Revolutionary Art of Happiness*

Nutrition, Creation, and Lifestyle Rhythms

Living in alignment with nature's design.

- **Ellen G. White** — *Ministry of Healing* (classic health and faith perspective)
- **Dr. Michael Klaper** — *True North Health* lectures and videos on fasting and restoration
- **Dan Buettner** — *The Blue Zones* (lessons from the world's healthiest communities)
- **Forest Bathing by Dr. Qing Li** — *The Japanese Art of Shinrin-Yoku*
- **Katherine May** — *Wintering* (the necessity of rest in life's seasons)
- **Thich Nhat Hanh** — *Peace Is Every Step* (presence in the everyday)

Community & Purpose

Building connection, meaning, and shared restoration.

- **Charles Eisenstein** — *The More Beautiful World Our Hearts Know Is Possible*
- **Parker J. Palmer** — *A Hidden Wholeness* (community and courage)
- **Howard Thurman** — *Meditations of the Heart*
- **Shasta Nelson** — *Friendships Don't Just Happen!* (creating healthy adult connection)
- **RISE Momentum Circle** — Join at www.healthyinheart.com/rise

For Further Exploration by Angel Tate Keaton

- *The Eden Way: Reclaiming Body, Mind, and Spirit Through the Creator's Original Design*
- *The Eden Journal Companion* — 49-day journey toward restoration
- *RISE: The 9 Pillars of Whole-Being Wellness* — coming soon

"Gather wisdom like wildflowers — some from science, some from spirit, and let them grow together until your life becomes a garden of balance." ~ *Angel Tate Keaton*

Appendix C: The RISE Framework Overview Chart

A Model for Whole-Being Wellness and Balanced Living

THE CORE PHILOSOPHY

RISE stands for Rooted, Intentional, Strong, and Energized — four interwoven dimensions of whole-being wellness. Each element builds on the next, creating a living circle of harmony for Mind, Body, Emotion, and Energy.

"When you live Rooted, act with Intention, grow Strong through grace, and stay Energized by alignment, you begin to live in rhythm with yourself."

THE CIRCLE OF BALANCE

The RISE Circle mirrors the interconnected nature of wellness. When one element falls out of harmony, all are affected — and healing one helps restore the others.

Mind — Body — Emotion — Energy

Balance is not symmetry. It is a conversation.
The goal is flow, not perfection.

Element	Essence	Restores	Focus Practices	Affirmation
Rooted	Stability in truth and grounded identity	*Mind & Spirit*	Grounding breath, nature walks, journaling "What anchors me?"	*"I am safe, seen, and supported."*
Intentional	Clarity in thought and choice	*Mind & Emotion*	Morning reflections, mindful transitions, conscious decision-making	*"I choose with awareness, not autopilot."*
Strong	Resilience through surrender and boundaries	*Body & Emotion*	Movement with meaning, emotional regulation, saying "no" with grace	*"I bend, but I do not break."*
Energized	Flow through alignment and joy	*Body & Spirit*	Nourishment, breathwork, creativity, honoring rest and play	*"I live in rhythm, not in rush."*

THE FOURFOLD RHYTHM OF RENEWAL

Each anchor expresses itself across time through recurring rhythms of restoration.

Cycle	Focus	Examples of RISE Practices
Daily Renewal	*Presence and nourishment*	Breathwork, gratitude journaling, mindful eating
Weekly Renewal	*Rest and reflection*	Sabbath pause, unplugging, community check-ins
Seasonal Renewal	*Adaptation and growth*	Aligning meals and movement to the season, decluttering, and re-evaluating commitments
Lifelong Renewal	*Legacy and evolution*	Living aligned with purpose, mentoring, storytelling, and leaving the world better than you found it

THE PATH OF TRANSFORMATION

Every journey toward balance moves through four stages — gently, cyclically, and at your own pace:

1. **Awareness** → Noticing what is out of balance
2. **Acceptance** → Acknowledging truth without shame
3. **Alignment** → Making conscious changes
4. **Embodiment** → Living what you now know

"Healing is not becoming someone new — it's remembering who you were before you forgot your wholeness."

THE RISE MANTRA

Rooted in truth.
Intentional in habits.
Strong in spirit.
Energized for the hope of tomorrow.

Stay in RISE.

Appendix D: How to Join the RISE Momentum Circle

If this book has stirred something inside you—a hunger for connection, accountability, or renewal—you don't have to walk this journey alone. You are invited to join the RISE Momentum Circle, a supportive community dedicated to living out the *Rooted, Intentional, Strong, and Energized* way of life.

What Is the RISE Momentum Circle?

The Momentum Circle is a safe, inclusive space where we practice whole-being wellness together. Each week, we meet online to explore one aspect of the *Nine Anchors* of wellness—body, mind, emotion, and spirit—and share real-life applications of the RISE rhythm.

It's not about perfection. It's about showing up, reflecting honestly, and growing together.

Inside the Circle, You'll Find:

- **Weekly Gatherings:** Guided conversations on whole-being wellness, practical balance, and emotional healing.
- **Shared Reflection:** We dive into five weekly discussion questions with honesty and openness, exploring whole-being wellness together through meaningful, vulnerable conversation.
- **Accountability & Encouragement:** A rhythm of support that helps you stay consistent on your wellness path.
- **A Safe Community:** Belief-inclusive, judgment-free, and rooted in compassion.

How to Join

1. Visit **https://healthyinheart.com/contact-me-about-r-i-s-e**
2. Submit the short form.
3. You'll receive your welcome email with meeting details, the current week's topic, and a link to our Zoom gathering.
4. Bring your journal, a cup of tea, and an open heart.

Meetings are held **every Thursday evening, 5:00–6:30 PM EST** via Zoom.

You belong here.
Whether you're taking your first step toward balance or continuing a lifelong journey of renewal, the RISE Momentum Circle will meet you where you are—and help you rise, one rhythm at a time.

"Healing happens in community, not isolation. When we rise together, we remember who we were always meant to be."

~ Angel Tate Keaton

Appendix E: The 9 Pillars of RISE

The Nine Pillars of Wholeness

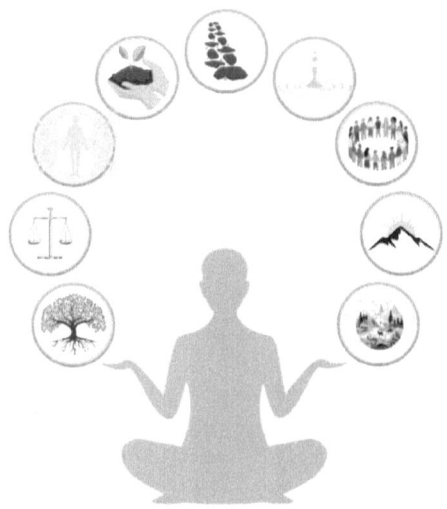

The pillars are listed in order. Each includes:

Symbol

Meaning

Daily practice focus

Reflection question

1. The Tree of Life — Rooted Health

Meaning: Connection, nourishment, vitality.

Wholeness begins underground: strong roots create strong lives.

Practice:

Eat from creation (living foods)

Move daily with gratitude

Rest before exhaustion

Reflection: What keeps my roots strong today?

2. The Scales of Balance — Living in Alignment

Meaning: Harmony across body, mind, spirit, and relationships.

Balance is alignment, not perfection.

Practice:

Pause mid-day to breathe and recenter

Simplify one crowded area

Reflection: Where can I recalibrate gently instead of striving?

3. The Radiant Human — Flowing Energy Within

Meaning: Inner light and vitality flow freely when beliefs, thoughts, and spirit agree.

Practice:

Begin with three deep breaths

Practice prayer, meditation, or mindful movement

Reflection: How can I let my inner light guide my pace?

4. Hands of Stewardship — Nurturing What's Given

Meaning: Responsibility, gratitude, and tending what has been entrusted.

Practice:

Do one act of care for your body, home, or relationships

Give encouragement or gratitude

Reflection: What am I stewarding with love today?

5. The Garden Path — Healing as a Journey

Meaning: Growth is not linear. Real healing bends, curves, and unfolds over time.

Practice:

Notice progress without judgment

Rest purposefully once a week

Reflection: What is today teaching me about patience?

6. The Water Ripple — The Power of Small Choices

Meaning: Every choice sends ripples into the whole system.

Practice:

Do one nourishing action

Notice its ripple through mood and relationships

Reflection: How can one small shift bring wider peace?

7. The Circle of People — Healing Together

Meaning: Belonging and connection are essential. We heal in community, not isolation.

Practice:

> Reach out to encourage someone

> Ask for help when needed

Reflection: Who forms my circle of support?

8. Sunrise Over Mountains — Renewal & Hope

Meaning: Dawn after darkness; every day is a new beginning.

Practice:

> Begin with gratitude

> Reframe setbacks as sunrise lessons

Reflection: Where do I see new light emerging?

9. The Heart in Creation — Love as the Core of Wholeness

Meaning: Love sustains the ecosystem of wellness — compassion, unity, and divine rhythm.

Practice:

Speak kindness to yourself and others

Do one act of care for creation

Reflection: How can I let love move through me today?

How the RISE Framework, Circle of Wholeness, and Nine Anchors Work Together

These three layers form a complete ecosystem:

RISE = the four qualities of a whole person

Rooted • Intentional • Strong • Energized

The Circle of Wholeness = the whole-life model

A dynamic view of alignment and balance,

where each area influences the others.

The Nine Anchors = the daily practices

Simple, repeatable habits that create sustainable balance over time.

Together, they help you:

Restore your sense of balance

Regulate your pace and internal rhythms

Smooth emotional edges

Establish nourishing routines

Develop steady energy

Live aligned with your values

Return to the Creator's design

Build a life that supports your wholeness

Appendix F: The Seven-Year RISE Journey

The Seven-Year RISE Journey is a long-form path of restoration, integration, and lived transformation. It is not a program to rush through or a system to master, but a framework to return to again and again as the seasons of life unfold.

Rooted in the RISE framework—Rooted, Intentional, Strong, Energized—this journey recognizes that real healing and wholeness do not happen in a single season. They unfold in cycles. Over seven years, participants move through repeated seasons of grounding, clarity, resilience, and renewal, allowing insight to mature into embodiment.

Each year builds upon the last, offering space to revisit familiar themes from deeper places of awareness. What begins as learning becomes practice. What begins as practice becomes pattern. And what becomes pattern eventually reshapes how you live, choose, rest, and relate—to your body, your boundaries, your faith, and your energy.

The Seven-Year RISE Journey honors the reality of being human. There is room for setbacks, pauses, grief, growth, and recalibration. Nothing is forced. Nothing is skipped. The work is gentle, honest, and cumulative.

Rather than asking you to become someone new, RISE invites you to return to what has always been true—steadily, patiently, and with compassion for the pace of real life.

This is not about quick fixes or constant self-improvement.

It is about learning how to live in balance—over time.

Acknowledgment of Sources

Throughout this book, I've referenced the work, wisdom, and research of many respected voices in the fields of psychology, medicine, spirituality, and holistic wellness.

All such references are used for educational and illustrative purposes to honor their contributions to the greater conversation around whole-being health.

Quotations and concepts are drawn from publicly available works by:

Dr. John McDougall, Dr. Caldwell Esselstyn, Dr. T. Colin Campbell, Dr. Neal Barnard, Dr. Doug Lisle, Dr. Alan Goldhammer, Dr. Caroline Leaf, Dr. Gabor Maté, Dr. Kristin Neff, BJ Fogg, Brené Brown, HeartMath Institute, and others listed in the *Resources & Recommended Reading* section.

Every effort has been made to give credit where due and to cite materials accurately. If any unintentional omission or oversight has occurred, it will be corrected in subsequent printings.

About the Author

Angel Tate Keaton is the founder of Healthy in Heart Media, LLC, a faith-rooted publishing and lifestyle brand devoted to restoring wholeness of body, mind, and spirit.

She is the creator of the RISE Whole-Being Wellness Framework and author of *The Eden Way* series, *RISE Wellness Journal*, and *Seeds of Truth Activity Book.* She coauthored with her husband, Todd G. Keaton, *The Little Keepers of the Garden: Seeds of Truth.*

A lifelong seeker of truth and wellness, Angel's journey began not in perfection but in pain. Raised in a strict Pentecostal Holiness home, she experienced early patterns of body shame, emotional suppression, abuse, and striving for approval. Years of chronic illness, disordered eating, and disconnection from her body eventually led her to question everything she had been taught about what it means to be "well."

Drawing on her background in psychology — where she earned her Associate of Arts and pursued her Bachelor of Science in Psychology — Angel blends academic insight with spiritual discernment to explore how belief, emotion, and behavior shape health. Her studies in cognition, trauma, and behavioral science deepened her conviction that true transformation begins in the mind but must flow through the body to become sustainable change.

Through the guidance of mentors who taught her to listen to the wisdom of the body and inspired her to seek truth without fear, Angel began rebuilding her life from the inside out. Along the way, she discovered the intersection between psychology, nutrition, and faith — and how healing begins when belief and biology come back into alignment.

Today, Angel writes and teaches about whole-being wellness, emotional integration, and the rhythm of sacred balance. She is a voice of hope for those walking out of perfectionism, trauma, and burnout into the peace of embodied living. Her work bridges modern health science with ancient Hebraic wisdom, reminding readers that true wellness is not achieved through striving but through remembering who we were created to be.

Through *Healthy in Heart Media*, Angel creates books, journals, devotionals, and children's series all centered around restoration, compassion, and connection with creation.

When she isn't writing, Angel can be found tending her garden, creating art, studying Scripture, or gathering with her communities in the RISE Momentum Circle and the Sabbath Table Gathering — a weekly space for shared reflection, encouragement, and whole-being growth.

Her message is simple:

"Healing isn't about becoming someone new. It's about returning to rhythm — and remembering that you were whole all along."

Also By Angel Tate Keaton

The Daniel Fast 21-Day Meal Plan: Simple Plant-Based Nourishment for Mind, Body & Spirit Eat Well. Pray Deep. Stand Strong.

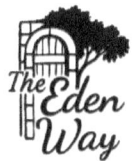

Books in the Series

B1----------- *The Eden Way*^{TM}*: Reclaiming Body, Mind, and Spirit Through the Creator's Original Design*

B2 ----------- *The Eden Way*^{TM} *Journal: 49-Days to Reset Body, Mind, and Spirit*

(Companion to Book 1)

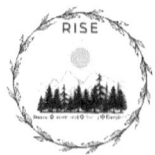

Books in the Series

RISE™ Wellness Journal—Rooted, Intentional, Strong, Energized: Embrace One Year of Habits, Healing, and Hope

RISE™ The Beginning of Balance—How Rooted, Intentional, Strong, and Energized Living Transforms the Whole Self: A Framework for Whole-Being Wellness

The Beginning of Balance Chronicles: The Lived Record of Learning to Inhabit RISE

The 9 Pillars of Whole-Being Wellness For A Balanced Life—A RISE^{TM} Guide to Realignment, Renewal, and Everyday Balance (Coming Soon)

The RISE™ 21 Seasons of Wholeness--A 7-Year Guided Rhythm (Coming Soon)

Identity & Worth Volume 1

RISE™ Identity & Worth Living a Rooted, Intentional, Strong, and Energized Life—Volume 1
RISE™ Identity & Worth Journal: A 12-Week Journey to a Rooted, Intentional, Strong, and Energized Life—Volume 1 (Companion to Identity & Worth, Volume 1)

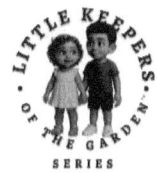

Books in the Series

The Little Keepers of the Garden^{TM}: Seeds of Truth Collection

Seeds of Truth Activity Book: The Little Keepers of the Garden^{TM} Series

The Little Keepers of the Garden^{TM}: The Keeper and the Garden's Gentle Rhythm (Coming Soon)

The Keeper and the Garden's Gentle Rhythm Activity Book: The Little Keepers of the Garden^{TM} (Coming Soon)

Scholarly Works

Righteousness Restored - Walking the Ancient Covenant Path of Jesus, Uncovering Paul's Impact on Law & Gospel (Coming June 2026)

If This Book Helped You Rise...

In the RISE rhythm, every step forward matters—every insight, every reflection, every moment of honesty.

If this book supported your journey toward a more rooted, intentional, strong, and energized life, I'd be honored if you would share your experience.

Your review isn't just feedback for my benefit. It becomes part of the circle—an encouragement to someone who may be standing right where you once stood, wondering if healing and balance are possible for them too.

You can leave a review here:

Goodreads

Amazon

HealthyInHeart.com

Thank you for showing up for yourself.

Thank you for rising.

And thank you for helping others discover a path to wholeness by sharing your voice.

.